Review of AIIMS

(November 2018)

AF530629

Celebrating 50 YEARS

Passion, Quality and Innovation in Healthcare Publishing

Review of AIIMS (November 2018)

By AIIMSonians, for future AIIMSonians

Gaurav Gupta
Senior Resident
Department of Medicine
AIIMS, New Delhi, India

Ankesh Gupta
Pursuing DM
(Infectious Diseases)
AIIMS, New Delhi, India
Rank 29 in AIIMS May 2018

JAYPEE

JAYPEE BROTHERS MEDICAL PUBLISHERS
The Health Sciences Publisher
New Delhi | London | Panama

Jaypee Brothers Medical Publishers (P) Ltd.

Headquarters

Jaypee Brothers Medical Publishers (P) Ltd
4838/24, Ansari Road, Daryaganj
New Delhi 110 002, India
Phone: +91-11-43574357
Fax: +91-11-43574314
E-mail: jaypee@jaypeebrothers.com

Overseas Offices

J.P. Medical Ltd
83, Victoria Street, London
SW1H 0HW (UK)
Phone: +44 20 3170 8910
Fax: +44 (0)20 3008 6180
E-mail: info@jpmedpub.com

Jaypee-Highlights Medical Publishers Inc
City of Knowledge, Bld. 235, 2nd Floor, Clayton
Panama City, Panama
Phone: +1 507-301-0496
Fax: +1 507-301-0499
E-mail: cservice@jphmedical.com

Jaypee Brothers Medical Publishers (P) Ltd
Bhotahity, Kathmandu, Nepal
Phone: +977-9741283608
E-mail: kathmandu@jaypeebrothers.com

Website: www.jaypeebrothers.com
Website: www.jaypeedigital.com

Inquiries for bulk sales may be solicited at: jaypee@jaypeebrothers.com

Review of AIIMS (November 2018)

First Edition: **2019**

ISBN: 978-93-5270-986-1

Printed at: Samrat Offset Pvt. Ltd.

Dedicated to

My mom-dad and
my brother Saurav

—Gaurav Gupta

Love of my life my mom-dad,
my God and Shweta

—Ankesh Gupta

CONTRIBUTORS

Amandeep Singh
Senior Resident
Department of Medicine
AIIMS, New Delhi, India

Antara DebBarma
Senior Resident
Department of Forensic Medicine
AIIMS, New Delhi, India

Ayush Goel
(Rank 2 AIIMS Nov 2018)
Junior Resident
Department of Medicine
AIIMS, New Delhi, India

Ishan Pandya
Junior Resident
Department of Ophthalmology
AIIMS, New Delhi, India

Kamna Choudhary
Junior Resident
Department of Pathology
RD Gardi, Medical College
Ujjain, Madhya Pradesh

Lina Barman
Junior Resident
Department of Pharmacology
AIIMS, New Delhi, India

Monalisa Sahu
Senior Resident
Infectious Disease
AIIMS, New Delhi, India

Nisha Tandon
(MBBS from JIPMER)
Junior Resident
Department of Otorhinolaryngology
AIIMS, New Delhi, India

Nizam
Junior Resident
Department of Microbiology
AIIMS, New Delhi, India

Pandu Chouhan
Senior Resident
Department of Pediatrics
AIIMS, New Delhi, India

Pankhuri Dudani
Department of Dermatology
AIIMS, New Delhi, India

Piyush Jaiswal
Department of Community Medicine
AIIMS, New Delhi

Prerna Singh
Ex Senior Resident
Department of Gynecology and Obstetrics
AIIMS, New Delhi, India

Radhika
(rank 2 AIIMS May 2018)
Junior resident
Department of Radio-diagnosis
AIIMS, New Delhi, India

Rajeev Gupta
Intern
AIIMS, New Delhi, India

Soumyadeep Chatterji
Senior Resident
Infectious Disease
Department of Medicine
AIIMS, New Delhi, India

Sourav Gupta
MBBS student
Gajar Raja Medical College
Gwalior, Madhya Pradesh, India

Umang Arora
(Rank 1 AIIMS Nov 2018)
Junior Resident
Department of Medicine
AIIMS, New Delhi, India

PREFACE

Being an AIIMSonians is the dream of every medical student. AIIMS is the apex institute of country and AIIMS entrance exam is among the toughest competitive exams. Questions in AIIMS entrance exam are mostly tricky. Apart from in-depth knowledge of all subjects, presence of mind during exam hours is essential. Knowledge of exam pattern and approach to solve AIIMS MCQ becomes imperative to secure good rank in AIIMS entrance exam as sometimes there is no correct answer but rather 3 incorrect answers.

We have worked hard to explain "why correct is correct and incorrect is incorrect".

This book is written by AIIMSonians. Repeated topics in AIIMS entrance exam are explained in detail with specific emphasis on those aspects which are common in our wards because of chances of appearance in future entrance is highly likely.

About AIIMS PG Entrance Exam

- 200 MCQs will decide your fate.
- Each correct answer gives 1 mark while wrong answer carries a negative marking of 1/3.
- **Minimum correct (approximately) 140/200 in November and 136/200 is required to achieve a rank within 100.**
- Going according to current trend of questions, 50-60 image-based, 2-5 video-based, 15-20 repeats (include topic repeat and similar question as in previous exam), expected sound-based questions (heart sound, respiratory auscultation) will appear in future entrance exams.
- Image based questions include ECGs, spot diagnosis, virus life cycle, one clinical scenario based parasitology, X-ray based questions (pneumothorax is AIIMS favorite), Trauma questions, Biostatistics which is very imp from AIIMS point of view.
- **Majority of questions are from repeat topics only**
- **Knowledge of all 4 options is essential.**

Gaurav Gupta
Ankesh Gupta

CONTENTS

ANATOMY

1. All of the following muscles help in inversion of foot *except*:

a. Tibialis posterior
b. Tibialis anterior
c. Peroneus longus
d. Extensor halluces longus

Ans. c. Peroneus longus

Inversion of the Foot

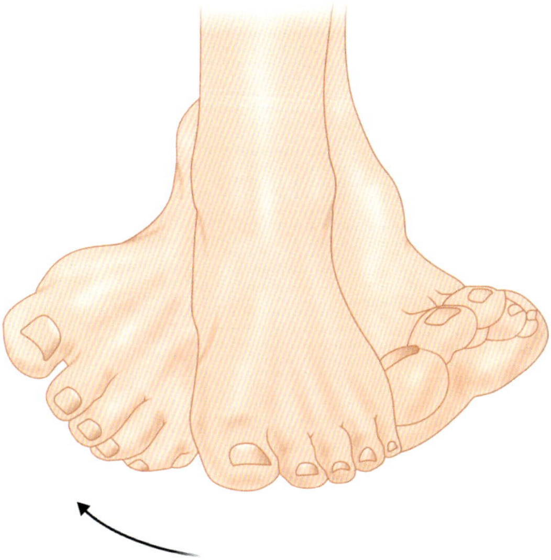

Inversion is a movement of the foot which causes the soles of the feet to face inwards, and eversion is the opposite movement.

Inversion and eversion occur primarily at:

- Talocalcaneonavicular joint
- Subtalar (talocalcaneal) joint

The muscles which cause inversion of the foot are:

- Tibialis anterior
- Tibialis posterior
- Extensor hallucis longus
- Triceps surae

2. Left superior intercostal vein drains into:

a. Hemi azygous vein
b. Brachiocephalic vein
c. Azygous vein
d. Internal thoracic vein

Ans. b. Brachiocephalic vein

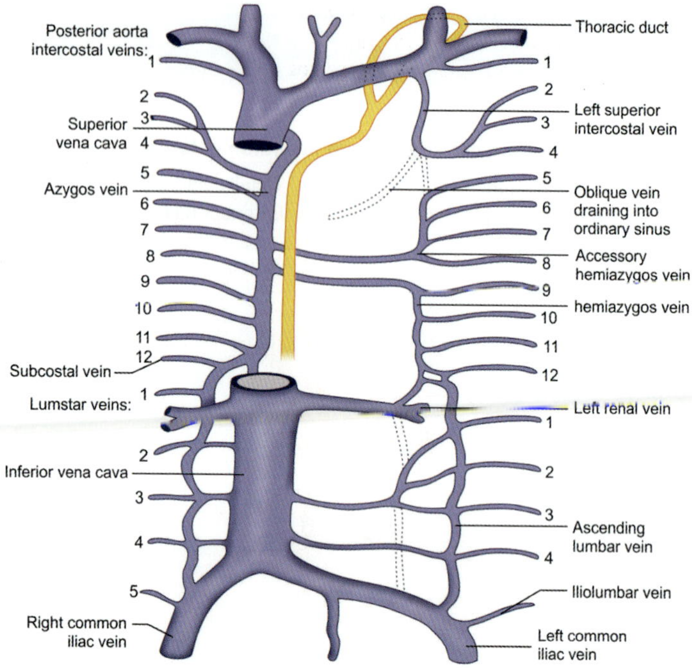

Intercostal Veins

- Two anterior intercostal veins and 1 posterior intercostal vein are included in every intercostal space

Anterior Intercostal Veins

- They are present only in the upper 9 spaces.
- Every space includes 2 veins and accompanies the anterior intercostal arteries.
- In upper 6 spaces, they stop in the internal thoracic vein.
- In seventh, eighth, and ninth spaces, they stop in the musculophrenic vein.

Posterior Intercostal Veins

- They are found in all the spaces.
- Every space includes only 1 posterior intercostal vein.
- Every vein accompanies the posterior intercostal artery.
- Its tributaries correspond to the branches of posterior intercostal artery.

Right Posterior Intercostal Veins

- 1st (highest) drains into the right brachiocephalic vein.
- 2nd, 3rd, and 4th join to form right superior intercostal vein, which in turn drains into the azygos vein.
- 5th–11th drain into the azygos vein.
- Subcostal vein drains into the azygos vein.

Left Posterior Intercostal Veins

- 1st (highest) drains into left brachiocephalic vein
- 2nd, 3rd, and 4th join to form left superior intercostal vein, which in turn drains into left brachiocephalic vein.

- 5th–8th drain into accessory azygos vein
- 9th-11th drain into hemiazygos vein.
- Subcostal vein drains into the hemiazygos vein.

3. What is the action of marked muscle in the given image?

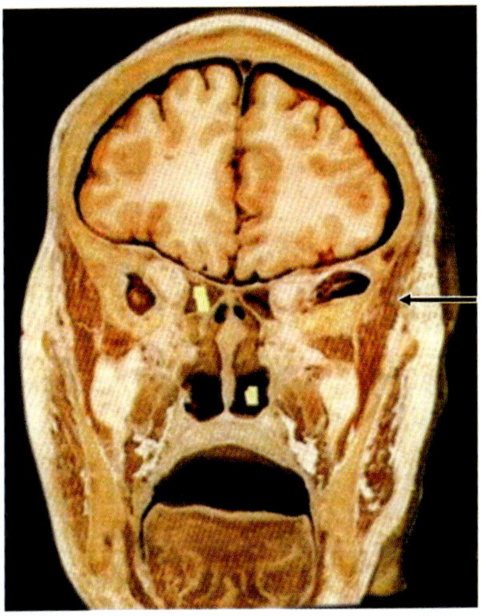

a. Elevation
b. Depression
c. Protraction
d. Retraction

Ans. a. Elevation

Marked Muscle is Temporalis

- Temporalis
  - It is connected above to the temporal line and below to the zygomatic arch and is covered by tough temporal fascia.
  - It is located in the temporal fossa and is a fan-shaped muscle.
- Origin
  It appears from:
  - Whole of the floor of temporal fossa with the exception of the part created by the zygomatic bone.
  - Deep surface of the temporal fascia.
- Insertion
  The fibers converge and descend to create a tendon, which goes through the gap between the zygomatic arch and the side of the skull. The muscle is added into:
  - The medial surface, apex, anterior, border of the coronoid process of ramus of mandible
  - The anterior border of the ramus of mandible, nearly up to the final molar tooth. The temporalis muscle is fan shaped. The anterior fibers are oriented vertically, the posterior-most fibers are disposed nearly horizontally and interceding intermediate fibers are positioned obliquely.
- Nerve supply
  - The temporalis is supplied by the anterior and posterior deep temporal nerves, the branches of the anterior section of the mandibular nerve.

Muscle	Superior attachment	Interior attachment	Function	Nerve supply
Masseter	Anterior twothirds of the inferior border of the zygomatic arch and the zygomatic process of the maxilla	Lower twothirds of the outer surface of the ramus of the mandible	Elevation some side to side movement and protrusion of the mandible	Masseter branch of the mandibular
Temporalls	Temporal fossa on the lateral surface of the skull and the temporals fascia	Superior margin of the coronoid process extending onto the ramus of the mandible	Elevation side to side movement and retraction of the mandible	Deep temporal branches of the mandibular
Medial pterygoid	Medial surface of the lateral ptergoid plate, and the adjacent palatine bone and maxillary tuberosity	Lower half of the medial surface of the ramus of the mandible	Elevation side to side movement and protrusion of the mandible	Medial pterygoid branch of the mandibular
Lateral pterygoid	Upper head: infratemporal surface of the greater wing of the sphenoid bone lower head: lateral surface of the lateral pterygoid plate	Neck of the mandible and the intra-articular disc of the temporo-mandibular joint	Side to side movement and protrusion of the mandible: acting together the two heads flatten the disc and open the mouth	Lateral pterygoid branch of the mandibular

4. All of the following bones are involves in wrist formations *except*:

a. Scaphoid
b. Ulna
c. Radius
d. Triquetral

Ans. b. Ulna

Wrist Joint (Radio-Carpal Joint)

- Radio-Carpal Joint is the wrist joint that lies in the middle of the lower end of radius and carpus.
- It is a synovial joint of ellipsoid variety.

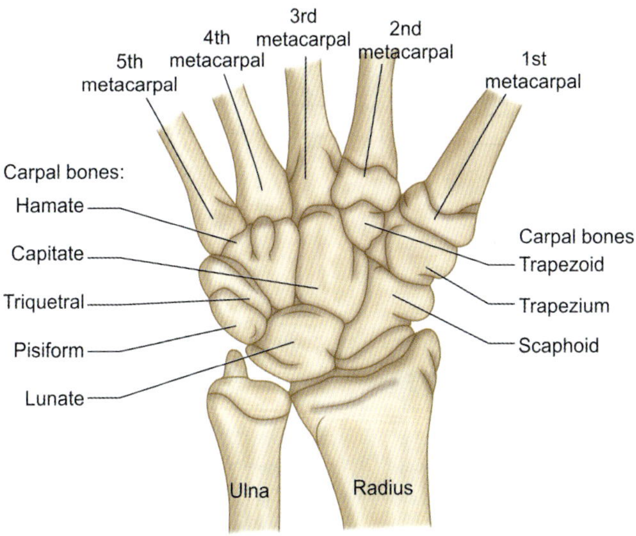

Articular Surfaces

- The inferior surface of the lower end of radius and inferior surface of the triangular articular disc of inferior radio-ulnar joint together forms Proximal articular surface.
- This proximal articular surface is concave from side to side and almost elliptical in shape
- Distal articular surface is formed by the proximal surfaces of scaphoid, triquetral, and lunate bones. It is smooth and convex.
- Although wrist joint is an articulation between forearm and hand, the medial bone of forearm — the ulna is excluded from this articulation by an articular disc.
- In the neutral position of the wrist, only the scaphoid and lunate are in contact with the radius and articular disc; the triquetral comes into contact with the articular disc only in the full adduction of the wrist.

5. Which of the following cranial nerve not associated with olfaction?

a. XII b. IX

c. V d. X

Ans. a. XII

Hypoglossal nerve is the 12th cranial nerve and originates from the medulla oblongata. It is a pure motor nerve

- Hypoglossal nerve is a motor nerve which, involved in the movement of tongue muscles, swallowing and speech.
- It innervates all the muscles of the tongue except palatoglossus muscle which is innervated by the vagus nerve.

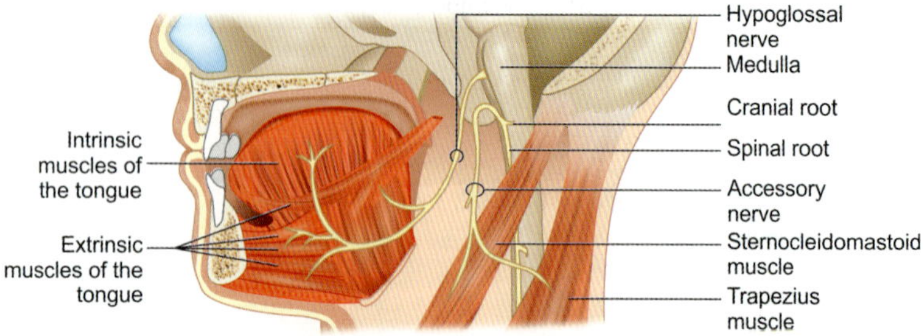

6. Occlusion of the artery supply marked area will cause all *except*:

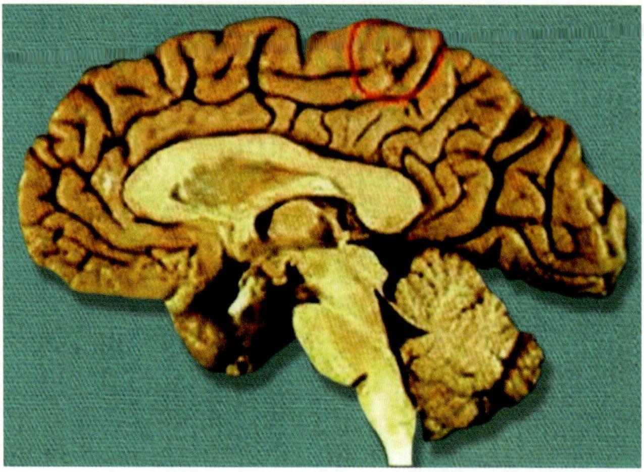

a. Urinary incontinence
b. Rectal incontinence
c. Apraxia
d. Perianal anesthesia

Ans. c. Apraxia

Marked area is paracentral lobule.

Paracentral Lobule

- Paracentral lobule is on the medial surface of the hemisphere and is the continuation of the precentral and postcentral gyri.
- The paracentral lobule controls motor and sensory innervations of the contralateral lower extremity.
- It is also responsible for control of defecation and urination.

7. Patient with syphilis develops imbalance on walking with eyes closed and has to lift up foot and stamp on ground to walk. Name the tract involved in given condition:

a. Spinocerebellar tract
b. Dorsal column tract
c. Lateral spinothalamic tract
d. Vestibulospinal tract

Ans. b. Dorsal column tract

Given condition represents Positive Romberg test

- In the Romberg test, the patient stands upright and asked to close his eyes. A loss of balance is interpreted as a positive Romberg sign.
- The Romberg test is used to demonstrate the effects of posterior column disease upon human upright postural control.
- Posterior column disease involves selective damaging of the posterior column, known as tabes dorsalis neurosyphilis.

8. Ligamentum flavum consists of:

a. Type-II collagen　　b. Type-I collagen
c. Reticulin　　d. Elastin

Ans. d. Elastin

Ligamentum Flavum

- The ligamentum flavum is a short but thick ligament that connects the laminae of adjacent vertebrae from C2 to S1.
- It consists of 80% elastin and 20% collagen.
- At each intersegmental level the ligamentum flavum is a paired structure being represented symmetrically on both sides.

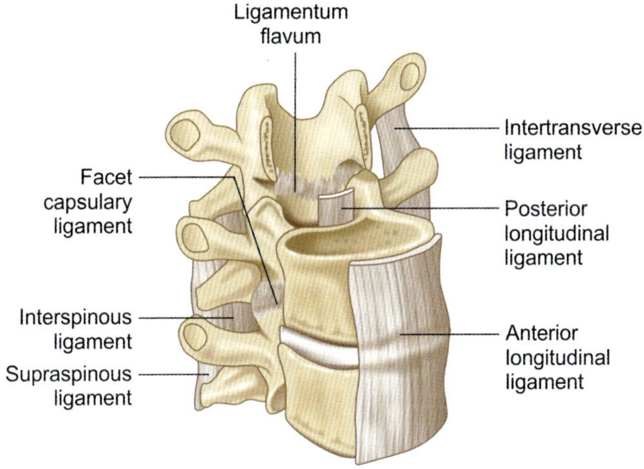

- Each includes yellow elastic tissue, the fibers which, nearly perpendicular in instructions, are connected to the anterior side of the lamina above, some distance via its inferior margin, and to the posterior side and upper margin of the lamina underneath.
- The ligamenta flava help to bring back the erect posture after flexion therefore guarding the disc via the injury and avoid the splitting up of laminae in spinal flexion.

9. Golgi apparatus in serous acinar cells is at:

a. Supranuclear　　b. Apical
c. Adjacent to nucleus　　d. Basal

Ans. a. Supranuclear

The Golgi apparatus is usually located midway along the cell, typically in a supranuclear position.

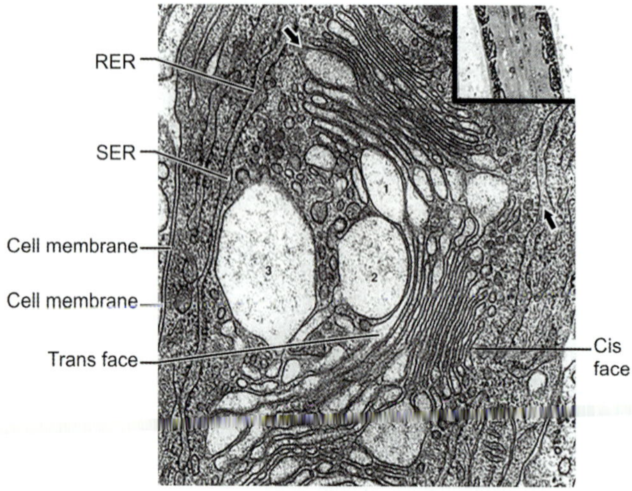

- Serous acinar cells are arranged in small acini of 5-10 cells with a very small central lumen.
- Each acinar cell is roughly pyramid-shaped, with its apex at the lumen.
- The cells basal ends contain the large rounded nuclei and an abundance of rough ER.
- A portion of one acinar cell is shown ultrastructurally, indicating the abundant RER, Golgi complexes, and secretory granules and the very small size of the acinus lumen.
- Secretion here is merocrine and typically the mature zymogen granules, filled with digestive enzymes, remain in the apical cell region until the cell is stimulated to secrete.
- Other cells secrete constitutively, with small granules undergoing exocytosis as soon as they emerge fully formed from the Golgi apparatus.

10. What is the location of Meissner's corpuscles?

a. Lucidum b. Basale
c. Reticular dermis d. Papillary dermis

Ans. d. Papillary dermis

The papillary region is composed of loose areolar connective tissue. This is named for its fingerlike projections called papillae, that extend toward the epidermis and contain either terminal networks of blood capillaries or tactile Meissner's corpuscles.

11. What is normally seen in lumbar spine?

a Scoliosis b. Lordosis
c. Kyphosis d. Recurvatum

Ans. b. Lordosis

- Normal lordosis is the two forward curves seen in the neck (cervical spine) and low back (lumbar spine)
- Normal kyphosis is the two backward curves seen in the chest (thoracic spine) and hip areas (sacral spine). Each of the naturally occurring and normal soft curves serves to distribute mechanical stress incurred as the body is at rest and during movement.

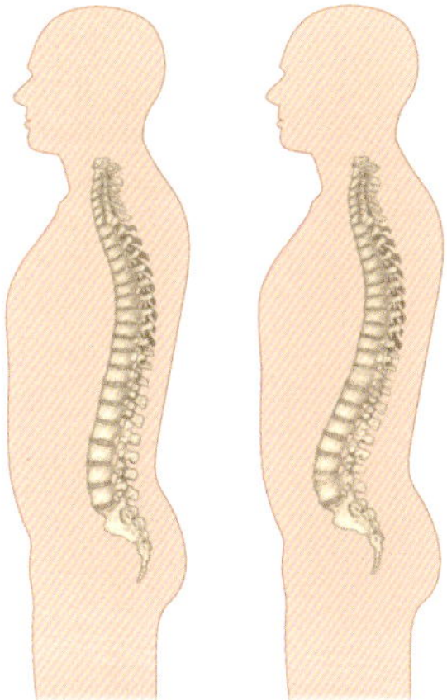

12. Identify the marked layer in the given histological section:

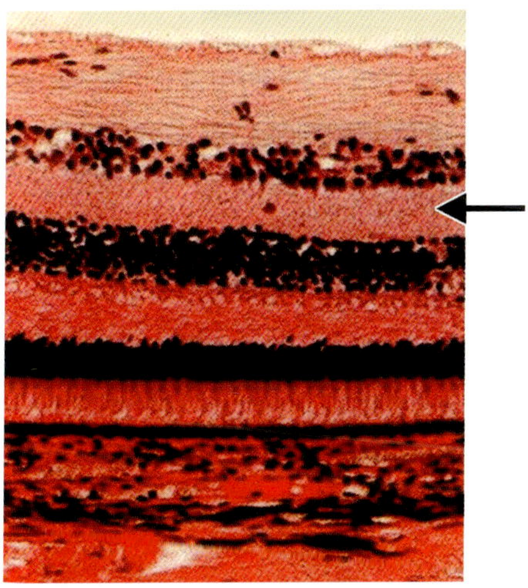

a. Inner plexiform layer
b. Outer plexiform layer
c. Inner limiting layer
d. Outer limiting layer

Ans. a. Inner plexiform layer

- The retina is arranged in different layers of cells, from Retinal Pigment Epithelium (RPE), Outer Nuclear Layer (ONL), Outer Plexiform Layer (OPL), Inner Nuclear Layer (INL), Inner Plexiform Layer (IPL), and ganglion cell layer.
- The retinal layer harbors five retinal neuronal cells, primarily, the rod-and cone photoreceptors, the Müller glia, the horizontal cell, the bipolar cell, the amacrine cell, and the Retinal Ganglion Cell (RGC). The arrow indicates the light transmission into the retina.

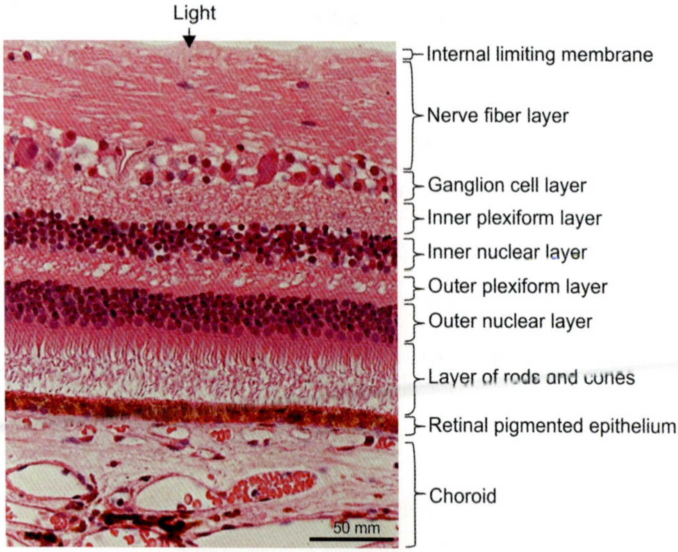

13. Identify the arrow marked nerve in the given section of cranial cavity:

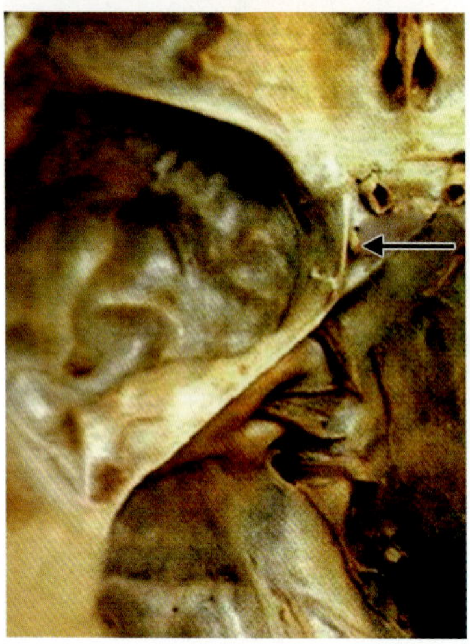

a. Trochlear
b. Trigeminal
c. Oculomotor
d. Abducent

Ans. c. Oculomotor

- Oculomotor nerve palsy or third nerve palsy is an eye condition resulting from damage to the third cranial nerve or a branch thereof.
- Oculomotor nerve supplies the majority of the muscles controlling eye movements.

Features of Occulomotor (3rd) Nerve Palsy

- Paralysis of superior rectus, inferior rectus, medial rectus and inferior oblique.
  - Eye is down and out due to unopposed action of superior oblique and lateral rectus.
  - Medial and upward gaze is not possible.
- Paralysis of sphincter pupillae→ Loss of ipsilateral direct and consensual pupillary light reflex and there is mydriasis.
- Paralysis of ciliary muscle→ Paralysis of accomodation and conversion reaction.
- Two extraocular muscles are spared
  - I. Superior oblique: Intorsion, abduction and depression remain active.
  - II. Lateral rectus: Abduction remains active. So eye is deviated laterally.
- Paralysis of levator palpebrae superioris→ Ptosis
- Oculomotor nerve is the most commonly involved cranial nerve in intracranial aneurysm.

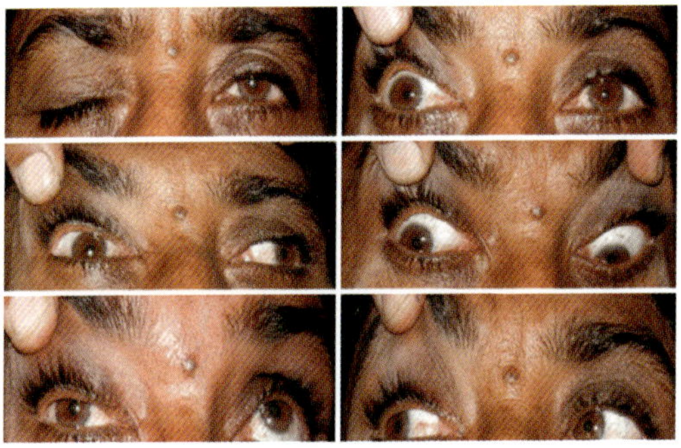

14. Type of connective tissue present in the arrow marked area is:

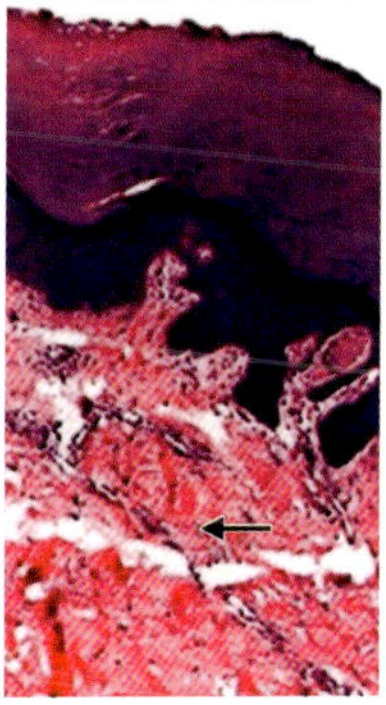

a. Loose and irregular
b. Specialized
c. Dense irregular
d. Dense regular

Ans. c. Dense irregular

Marked area in image is reticular dermis

- The reticular dermis is the lower layer of the dermis, found under the papillary dermis, composed of dense irregular connective tissue featuring densely packed collagen fibers.

- It is the primary location of dermal elastic fibers.

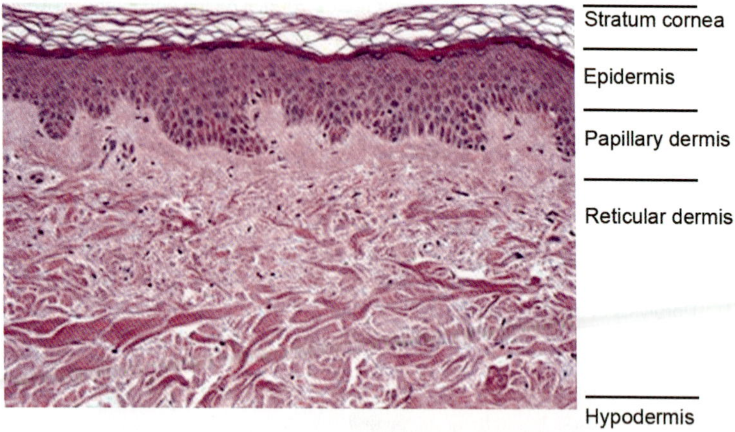

15. Correct pairing regarding between lymph node and their anatomical boundaries is:

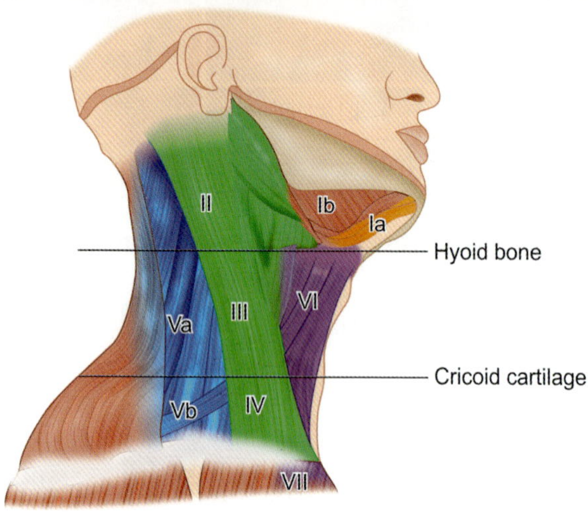

a. **Level 5**: Base of skull to cricoid
b. **Level 4**: Hyoid to cricoid
c. **Level 6**: Hyoid to clavicle
d. **Level 3**: Cricoid to clavicle

Ans. c. Level 6: Hyoid to clavicle

Classification of lymph nodes of neck or cervical lymph nodes based on American Academy of Otolaryngology and the American Joint Committee on Cancer

Level 1

- Inferior towards mylohyoid muscle and superior towards the lower border of the hyoid bone or the carotid division.
- Anterior towards the posterior boundary of the submandibular glands.

Level I: (a) Submental nodes.

Level I: (b) Submandibular nodes.

Level II:

- Internal jugular a.k.a. deep cervical chain.
- Base of the skull towards the inferior margin of hyoid bone or the carotid division.
- Anterior towards the posterior rim of sternocleidomastoid muscle.
- Posterior towards the posterior rim of the submandibular glands.

Level II: (a) Anterior, lateral, medial, or posterior towards the internal jugular vein.

- Most superior node is the jugulodigastric node.

Level II: (b) Posterior towards the internal jugular vein and have a fat layer dividing the nodes as well as the vein.

Level III

- Internal jugular a.k.a. deep cervical chain.
- Lower margin of hyoid towards lower border of cricoid cartilage or the middle tendon of omohyoid.
- Anterior towards the posterior border of sternocleidomastoid muscle.
- Lateral towards the medial margin of the common carotid artery/internal carotid artery.

Level IV

- Internal jugular or deep cervical chain.
- Lower boundary of cricoid cartilage towards level of the clavicle.
- Anterior and medial towards an oblique line drawn via the posterior edge of sternocleidomastoid and the posterolateral margin of the anterior scalene muscle.
- Laterally to the medial margin of the common carotid artery.

Level V

- Posterior triangle or spinal accessory nodes.
- Posterior towards the back of the sternocleidomastoid muscle and anterior towards the trapezius muscle

Level V: (a) Superior half, posterior to levels II and III.
(b) Inferior half, posterior to level IV.

Level VI

- Prelaryngeal (Delphian node)/pretracheal
- Anterior towards visceral space.
- From the inferior margin of hyoid bone till the manubrium.
- Anterior towards levels III and IV.

Level VII

- Superior mediastinal nodes
- In the middle of common carotid artery, inferior to superior part of manubrium towards level of the brachiocephalic vein.

PHYSIOLOGY

1. Calculate net filtration with the following data:

P_{GC} = 42 mm Hg

π_{GC} = 12 mm Hg

P_{BC} = 16 mm Hg

Assume that no proteins were filtered.

a. 34 mm Hg
b. Data not sufficient
c. 14 mm Hg
d. 28 mm Hg

Ans. c. 14 mm Hg

$P_{UF} = P_{GC} - P_T - \pi_{GC}$

P_{CO} = Hydrostatic pressure

π_{GC} = Osmotic pressure

P_T = Pressure in Bowman's capsule

P_{UF} = Filtration fraction

2. Hormones which is/are under inhibitory control of hypothalamus:

a. Prolactin
b. Prolactin only
c. GH
d. Both GH and prolactin

Ans. d. Both GH and Prolactin

Ref: Ganong 25th edition pg 324-331

- The hypothalamus controls growth hormone production by secreting growth hormone–releasing hormone (GHRH) which inhibits growth hormone release.
- Prolactin production is inhibited by **Prolactin inhibiting harmone (similar to Dopamine)** secreted by hypothalamus, which inturn inhibit prolactin.

3. Which hormone has permissive role is puberty?

a. Leptin
b. GnRH
c. Insulin
d. GH

Ans. a. Leptin

Ref: Ganong 25th edition Pg. 397

- It has been argued for some time that a critical body weight must normally be reached for puberty to occur. Thus, for example, young women who engage in strenuous athletics lose weight and stop menstruating, as do girls with anorexia nervosa. If these girls start to eat and gain weight, they menstruate again, that is, they "go back through puberty."
- It now appears that leptin, the satiety-producing hormone secreted by fat cells, may be the link between body weight and puberty. However, the way that leptin fits into the overall control of puberty remains to be determined.

4. Erythropoietin acts on:

a. CFU
b. Late erythroblast
c. Normoblast
d. Burst forming unit (BFU)

Ans. a > d. CFU > BFU

Ref: N Geetha Text book physiology pg. 79

- CFU E is sensitive to EPO (which decreases as the cells mature). CFU E contains highest density of erythropoietin receptors on their membrane and they depend on EPO for their survival
- BFU also require EPO only during its later stages of development

5. Which of the following heart sound may be a normal finding during pregnancy?

a. Fixed splitting of S2 b. S3
c. S4 d. Pericardial knock

Ans. b. S3

Ref: 24th edition William Obstetrics pg 59

Many of the normal cardiac sounds are modified during pregnancy.

- Splitting of first heart sound and increased loudness of both components
- No change in second heart sound (both aortic and Pulmonary element)
- Loud and easily heard third heart sound
- Systolic murmur intensified during inspiration which disappear shortly after delivery (in 90% of pregnant women)
- Soft diastolic murmur (in 20% of population)
- Continuous murmur in about 10 % of pregnant women

6. Integrin connects actin to which macromolecule in ECM?

a. Laminin b. Collagen
c. Fibronectin d. Vitronectin

Ans. c. Fibronectin

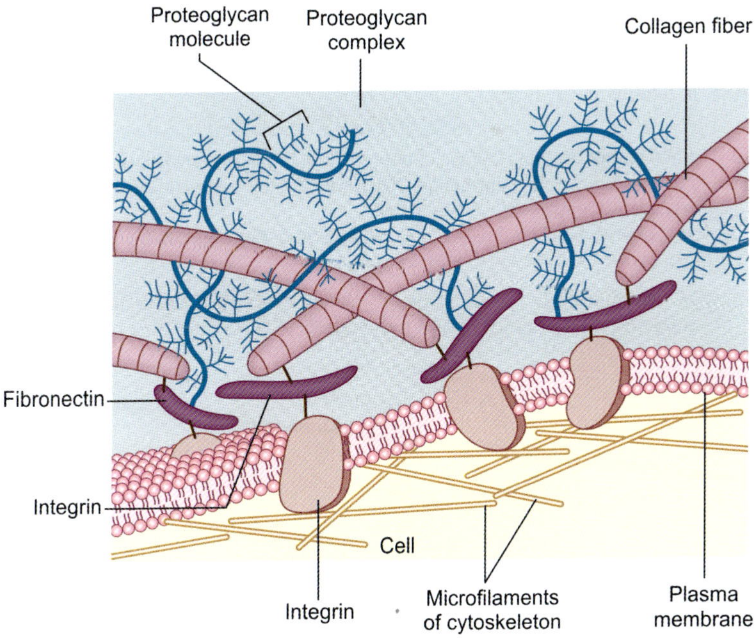

7. Which cell organelle is absent in cardiac muscle in the region marked by arrow?

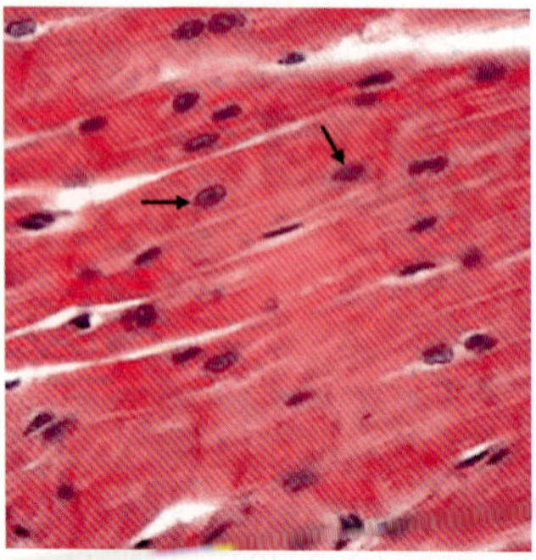

a. Mitochondria
b. Golgi body
c. SER
d. Lysosome

Ans. d. Lysosome

Ref: Ganong's Review of medical physiology 25th edn. page no. 112

- The marking areas are centrally placed nuclei
- The single nucleus of the cardiac muscle cell is located in the centre of the cell.
- Myofibril pass around the nucleus, producing a biconical juxtanuclear region in which the other organelles are concentrated.
- This perinuclear region is rich in mitochondria and contains a Golgi apparatus, glycogen granules, and lipofuscin granules.

8. Fibers reaching directly to Purkinje cell of cerebellum arise from which of the following?

a. Vestibular nucleus
b. Inferior olivary nucleus
c. Raphe nucleus
d. Locus ceruleus

Ans. b. Inferior olivary nucleus

Ref: RI Bijlani and Manjunatha text book of Physio

- White matter contains 2 types of afferent fibers (i) Mossy and (ii) climbing fibers
- Climbing fibers bring information ONLY from inferior olivary nuclei and establish excitatory synapse with Pukinje cells
- Rest of the input from the cerebellum are brought by other fibers called mossy fibers which synapse with granule cells

9. In the histology section given, which marked area is involved in relieving pain in response to massage?

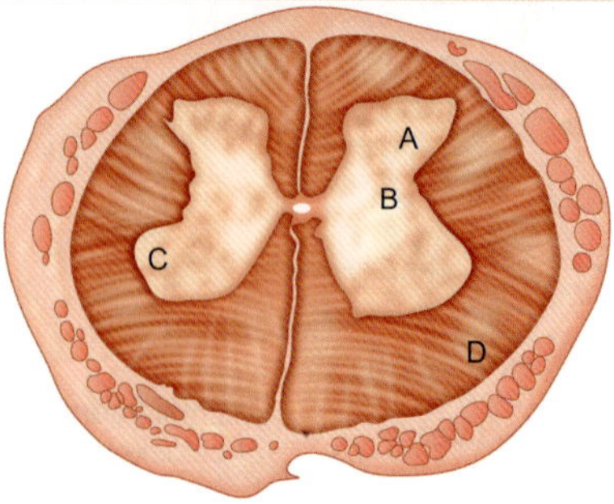

a. A
b. B
c. C
d. D

Ans. a. A

"Mezack and Wall" gate control theory of pain

- Massage stimulates A-beta fiber, which acts on gelatinosa neurone (G neuron) of dorsal of spinal cord.
- G neuron in turn inhibits small diameter pain fiber (closing the gate at spinal cord level.

10. Weber-Fechner law related to:

a. Number of nerves fiber
b. Number of muscles fiber
c. Number of stimulus
d. Intensity of stimulus

Ans. d. Intensity of stimulus.

Weber Fechner law states that the magnitude of sensation felt is propionate to the logarithm of intensity of stimulus.

$S = K \times \log I$

S: Perceived stimulus intensity

k: Weber fraction

11. Maximum area in homunculus signifies:

a. Low control and skilled movements
b. More muscle fibers are present
c. Increased precisiveness of movements
d. None of the above

Ans. c. Increased precisiveness of movements

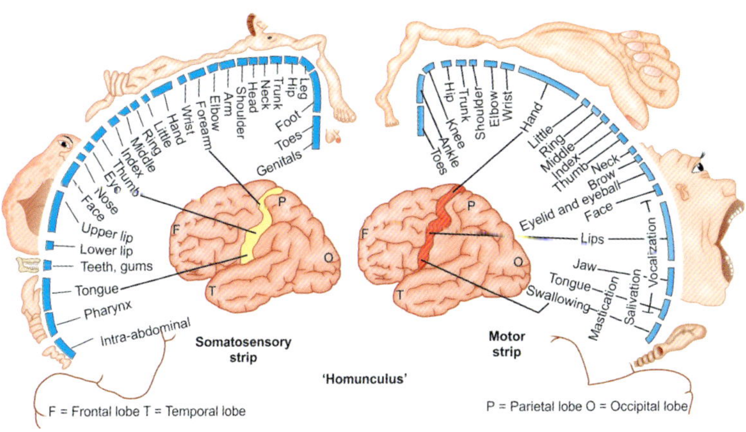

- In homunculus the largest areas represent the face, hands, and fingers, where precise localization is most important
- In homunculus the size of the various parts is proportionate to the use of the part skilled fine movement with precision.

12. Compliance curve of the lung given below: Curve A signifies which of the following?

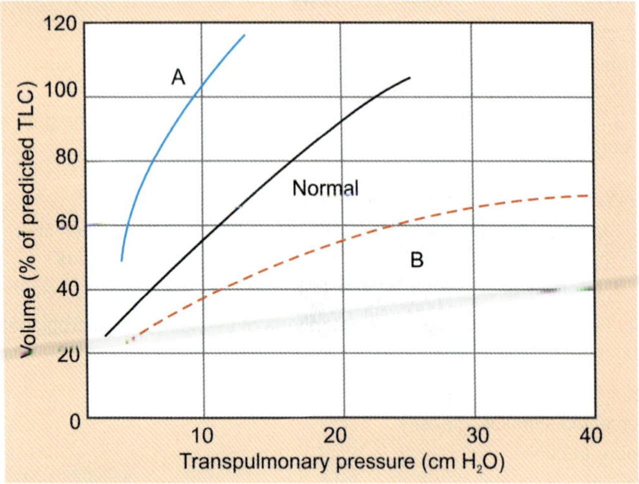

a. Pulmonary fibrosis
b. Atelectasis
c. Emphysema
d. ARDS

Ans c. Emphysmea

- A in the graph indicate increased compliance as seen in emphysema
- B in the graph indicate decreased compliance seen in pulmonary edema and interstitial pulmonary fibrosis.

BIOCHEMISTRY

1. Respiratory quotient after heavy carbohydrate meal is:

a. 1 b. 1.2

c. 0.8 d. 0.7

Ans. a. 1

- RQ = CO_2 eliminated / O_2 consumed
- The molecular formula, $C_6H_{12}O_6$, the complete oxidation equation is $C_6H_{12}O_6 + 6O_2 \rightarrow 6\ CO_2 + 6\ H_2O$. Thus, the RQ= 6 CO_2/6 O_2 = 1.

	CO_2 produced (L/S)	Q_2 consumed (L/g)	RQ
Carbohydrate	0.829	0.829	1.00
Protein	0.782	0.966	0.81
Fat	1.427	2.016	0.71
Alcohol	0.966	1.429	0.66

2. In noncompetitive antagonism which of the following is correct?

a. K_m decreases

b. No change in V_{max}

c. V_{max} decreases

d. Both K_m and V_{max} increases

Ans. c. V_{max} decreases

- The rate of an enzyme-catalyzed reaction increases with substrate concentration until a maximal velocity (V_{max}) is reached.
- Noncompetitive inhibition cannot be overcome by increasing the concentration of substrate.
- Thus, noncompetitive inhibitors decrease the apparent V_{max} of the reaction.

Competitive inhibition	Noncompetitive inhibition
It is reversed by increasing substrate concentration	Irreversible
Excess substrate abolishes inhibition	Excess substrate does not abolish the inhibition
V_{max} remains he same, but the apparent K_m is increased	**K_m remains the same, but the apparent V_{max} is decreased**
Inhibitor will be structural analogue of substrate	Inhibitors have no structural resemblance to substrate

3. During exercise, most rapid way to synthesize ATP is:

a. Glycogenolysis b. Glycolysis

c. TCA cycle d. Phosphocreatine

Ans. d. Phosphocreatine

- Phosphocreatine, also known as creatine phosphate (CP) or PCr (Pcr)
- It is a phosphorylated creatine molecule that serves as a rapidly mobilizable reserve of high energy phosphates in skeletal muscle and the brain to recycle adenosine triphosphate, the energy currency of the cell.
- Non-phosphorylated creatine is transformed into phosphocreatine by the enzyme complex creatine kinase, which makes it able to donate its phosphate group to convert adenosine diphosphate (ADP) into adenosine triphosphate (ATP).

4. In a child with cerebrohepatorenal syndrome and with hypotonia and hepatomegaly, the probable biochemical defect is accumulation of:

a. Pyruvate
b. Short-chain fatty acid
c. Very long-chain fatty acid
d. Acetyl CoA

Ans. c. Very long-chain fatty acid

- Zellweger syndrome, also called cerebrohepatorenal syndrome, is a rare congenital disorder characterized by the reduction or absence of functional peroxisomes in the cells of an individual.
- Caused by mutations in genes that encode peroxins, proteins required for the normal assembly of peroxisomes
- Patients have mutations that inactivate or greatly reduce the activity of both the maternal and paternal copies of one these aforementioned PEX genes.
- Impaired peroxisome function, an individual's tissues and cells can accumulate very long chain fatty acids (VLCFA) and branched chain fatty acids (BCFA) that are normally degraded in peroxisomes.

5. Patient with Type 1 diabetes mellitus, with complains of polyuria. Which of the following will occur normally in his body?

a. Glycogenesis in muscle
b. Increased conversion of fatty acid to acetyl CoA
c. Increased protein synthesis
d. Decreased cholesterol synthesis

Ans. b. Increased conversion of fatty acid to acetyl CoA

- In Type 1 diabetes mellitus, the onset of the disease is sudden, which is why the body switches abruptly from glucose utilization to fatty acid oxidation for energy needs.
- Acetyl CoA resulting from excess fatty acid oxidation saturates TCA cycle and the other alternative pathways resulting in ketogenesis
- Acetone, acetoacetate and β-hydroxybutyrate are the three ketone bodies formed

6. Northern blot is for:

a. Protein
b. DNA
c. RNA
d. DNA Protein interaction

Ans. c. RNA

- It is used to study gene expression by detection of RNA (or isolated mRNA) in a sample.
- With northern blotting it is possible to observe cellular control over structure and function by determining the particular gene expression rates during differentiation and morphogenesis.
- The term 'northern blot' actually refers specifically to the capillary transfer of RNA from the electrophoresis gel to the blotting membrane.

- Mnemonic: SNoW DRoP
  - S(southern) → D (DNA)
  - N (northern)→ R (RNA)
  - o → o
  - W (western)→ P (Protein)

7. Biomarker of alcoholic hepatitis are all *except*:

a. ALP b. AST
c. LDH d. GGT

Ans. c. LDH

- Alcoholic hepatitis (AH) is caused by acute inflammation of the liver in patients that consume excessive amounts of alcohol.
- While measurements of liver enzyme activities (GGT, ALT, AST) are important screening tools for detecting liver disease.
- Ethanol consumption behind hepatotoxicity may be obtained through measurements of blood ethanol and its specific metabolites (ethyl glucuronide, phosphatidylethanol, protein acetaldehyde condensates and associated autoimmune responses

8. Method of transport of glucose in the intestine is:

a. Primary active transport b. Secondary active transport
c. Simple diffusion d. Counter transport

Ans. b. Secondary active transport

- Glucose is absorbed in small intestine by absorptive cells.
- In secondary active transport, also known as coupled transport or co-transport, energy is used to transport molecules across a membrane.
- This energy comes from the electrochemical gradient created by pumping ions out of the cell
- Tho duodenum and upper jejunum absorb the bulk of the dietary sugars.
- Galactose and glucose are transported into the mucosal cells by an active, energy-requiring process that requires a concurrent uptake of sodium ions; the transport protein is the sodium dependent glucose cotransporter 1 (SGLT-1).

PATHOLOGY

1. How will you differentiate a mediastinal mass being a thymoma or ALL?

a. Cytokeratin b. CD1a.
c. CD3 d. Tdt

Ans. a. Cytokeratin

Cytokeratin is an epithelial cell marker (absent in lymphoma)
CD 1A Ia is positive for Langerhans cells and thymic lymphocytes and can be positive in some lymphomas
CD3: Single transduction complement of T-cells

Common all markers are:

BALL– TdT, CD22, CD10
TALL– TdT, CD2, CD5, CD4, CD8

	Thymoma	ALL
Cytokeratin	Present	Absent
Pax 8	Present	Absent
CD 1a	Present	Present
CD 99	Present	Present
Leucocyte common antigen	Present	Present

2. Which of the following tubes contain Sodium fluoride as anticoagulant?

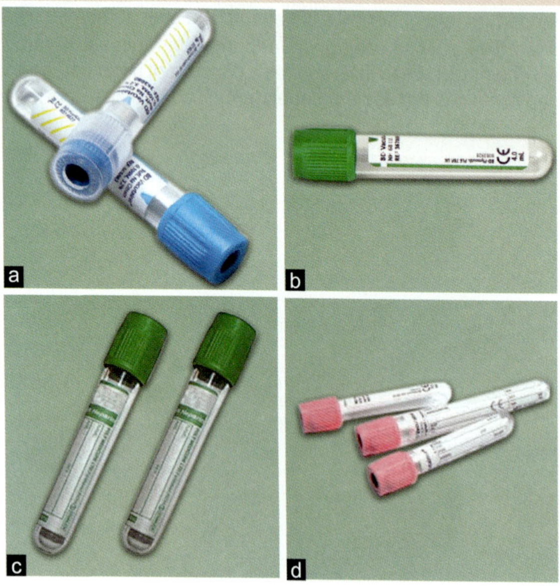

Ans. c.

Sodium fluoride is used as or anticoagulant. Answer is (c) grey vial

	Colour	Use	Anticoagulant
1.	Yellow vial	Blood culture	Sodium polyethanol sulfonate
2.	Light blue	Coagulation studies	Sodium citrate
3.	Red (plain vial)	Serum chemistries	No anticoagulant
4.	Green	Chemistry, osmotic fragility	Heparin
5.	Violet	CBC (Hematological studies	EDTA
6.	Grey	Blood glucose	Fluoride oxalate

3. Identify the inheritance pattern in the given pedigree:

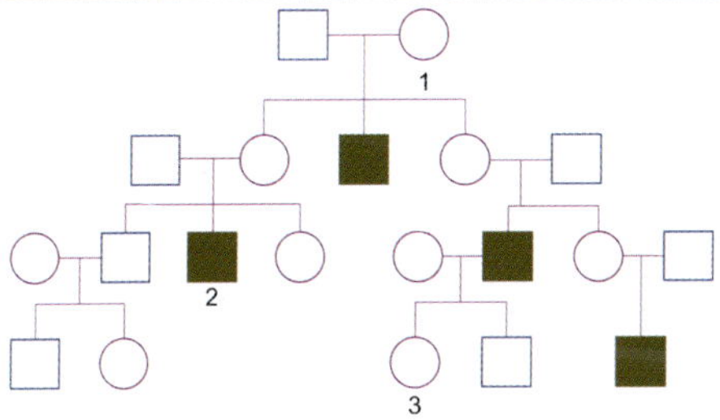

a. Y linked recessive
b. Y linked dominant
c. X linked recessive
d. X linked dominant

Ans. c. X linked recessive

- **X linked recessive:** Because it is not expressed in female population.
- Only expressed in male, absent in all fathers of male child because X chromosome comes from mother in case of male child.
- X linked recessive traits occurs much more frequently among males, because males are hemizygous.
- A female would express a recessive X linked trait only if she were homozygous recessive at that locus.
- All affected fathers transmit the recessive allele to all daughters and to none of their sons.
- Father to son transfer does not occurs
- All mothers of affected male child here is carrier of one defective X chromosome.

Why not...

- **X linked dominant**: Male with this trait passes it on to all his daughters and none of his sons.
- A female with the trait may passes it on to both her daughters and her sons
- Every affected person has at least one parent with the trait
- All the generations of pedigree is affected.

4. Naive T-cell get activated by:

a. NK cell
b. Dendritic cell
c. Macrophage
d. B-lymphocyte

Ans. b. Dendritic cell

Dendritic cells are the most potent stimulator of Naive T cells.

On coming in contact with antigen

- MHC & Manophage + antigen →determine whether invading antigen to presented to Br T lymphocytes
- Some strong antigens that cannot be dealt by antibody response from B cells like viruses, M.T.B., M. leprae, cancer cells, tissue transplantation antigen are presented to T cells.
- These specialized macrophages are called as antigen presenting cells, e.g. dendritic cells is lymphoid tissue and Langerhans cells in the epidermis.

5. A patient presented with intermittent fever, no weight loss, no anorexia, but with a retroperitoneal mass. Peripheral smear findings were normal. Gross & microscopy of the mass is given. What's the diagnosis?

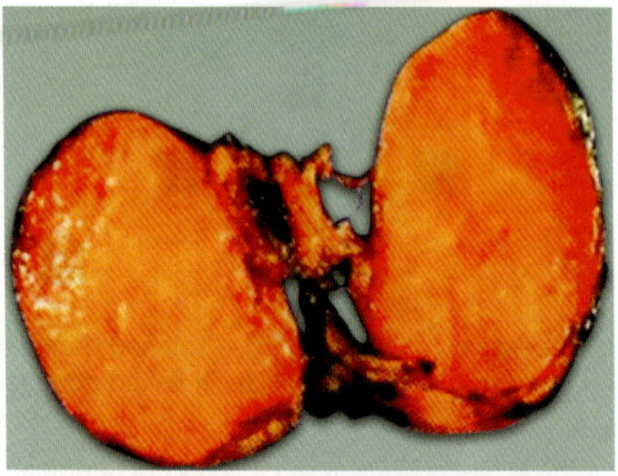

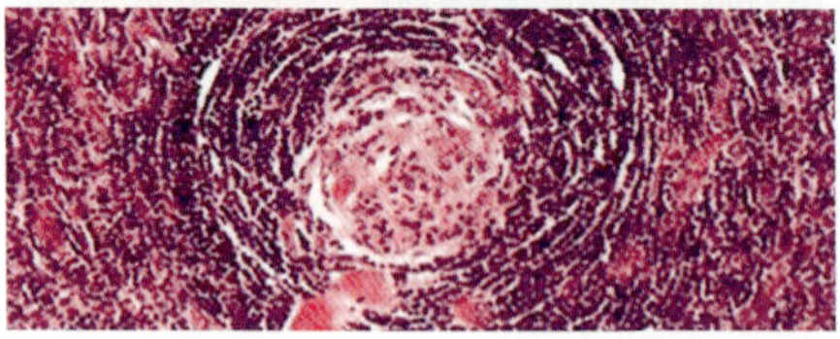

a. NHL
b. Castleman disease
c. Angiolymphoid hyperplasia
d. Ig G4 disease

Ans. b. Castleman disease

- Gross→Enlarged lymph node
- On cut tan-pink tissue with clarifications
- 3 variants
  - Hyaline vascular
  - Plasma cell type
  - Mixed hyaline vascular plasma cell

Clinical Presentation

- Hyaline vascular→solitary mass
- Plasma cell→solitary mass, fever, night sweats, fatigue weight loss, splenomegaly, anemia
- Mixed hyaline vascular plasma cell→All the above features including cytopenia, hypoalbuminemia
  Caused by HHV 8 infection is HIV patients

Microscopy

- Hyaline vascular
    - Prominent vascular proliferation and hyalinisation of vessel walls
    - 'Onion skin appearance' of mantle zones, (thickened mantle zones with lymphocytes arranged is layers)
    - Penetration of vessels in the germinal centres—Lollipop follicles
    - Extensive vascular proliferation with perivascular hyalinization in interfollicular areas.

Plasma Cell Variant

- Aggregates of lymph nodes with sheets of mature plasma cells in interfollicular areas.
- Hyperplastic germinal centres in follicles
- Plasma cell infiltrates in the intrafollicular areas.
- Multicentric/Mixed variant→Mix histological features of beta plasma cell & vascular hyaline.

6. Macrophage engulfs different cells as shown in the image, the process is called:

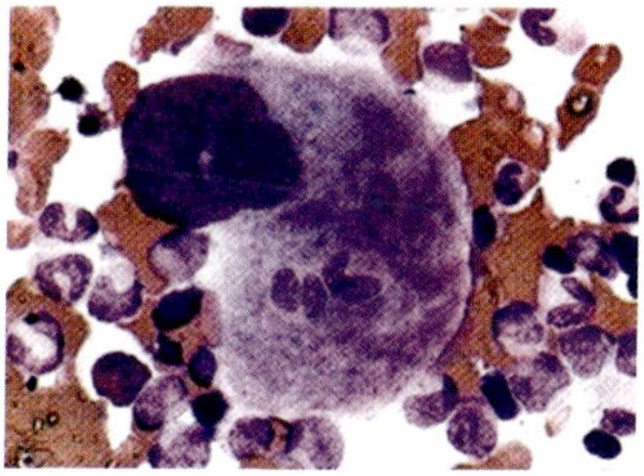

a. Phagocytosis
b. Emperipolesis
c. Killing
d. Cytotoxicity

Ans. b. Emperipolesis

Emperipolesis: Defined as active penetration of one cell by another which remains intact

Phagocytosis: Cell eating (engulfment of solid particulate material by cell).

Three ways:

- Recognition and attachment
- Engulfment
- Killing and degradation

Emperipolesis	Phagocytosis
Engulfed cell exists temporarily within another cell and with an intact normal structure	Engulfed cells is destroyed by lysosomal enzymes

7. Which is false about apoptosis?

a. No inflammation
b. Plasma membrane intact
c. Cellular swelling
d. Affected by dedicated genes

Ans. c. Cellular swelling

In apoptosis there is cell shrinkage not swelling.

Features of necrosis and apoptosis		
Feature	**Necrosis**	**Apoptosis**
Cell size	Enlarged (swelling)	Reduced (shrinkage)
Nucleus	Pyknosis → karyorrhexis → karyolysis	Fragmentation into nucleosome-size fragments
Plasma membrane	Disrupted	Intact; altered structure, especially orientation of lipids
Cellular contents	Enzymatic digestion; may leak out of cell	Intact; may be released in apoptotic bodies
Adjacent inflammation	Frequent	No
Physiologic or pathologic role	Invariably pathologic (culmination of irreversible cell injury)	Often physiologic, means of eliminating unwanted cells; may be pathologic after some forms of cell injury, especially DNA damage

8. A patient comes with chronic diarrhea with normal D-xylose test & abnormal schilling test. Duodenal biopsy is normal. What is the probable diagnosis?

a. Celiac disease
b. Ulcerative colitis
c. Ileal disease
d. Intestinal lymphangiectasia

Ans. c. Ileal disease

- *Illeum:* Vit. B_{12} absorption site.
- Schilling test is used for detection of Vit B_{12} malabsorption. Hence, abnormal schilling test indicates Vit B_{12} malabsorption i.e. illeal disease.
- D-Xylose test used for carbohydrate malabsorption, to it will be abnormal in malabsorption syndromes.
- Intestinal biopsy will be abnormal is conditions the coeliac disease, ulcerative colitis Crohn's disease. Tropical sprue, lymphangiectasia (congested and dilated lymphatic space)

9. A trauma patient presents at emergency department. There is no time for cross matching. FFP of which group can be transfused safely:

a. O Rh D+
b. O Rh D–
c. AB Rh D+
d. AB Rh D–

Ans. c. AB Rh D+

Landsteiner's Law

Blood group	Antigen	Antibody
A	A	Anti-B
B	B	Anti-A
AB	AB	Nil
O	Nil	Anti-A & anti-B

Answer is 'AB' positive FFP

- FFP plasma—Has few antibodies (mild variant of antibodies)
- 'AB' group—Has No antibodies only antigens
- Rh 'Positive'— Has No antibodies only antigens
- Hence, can be transfused safely

Whereas in case of blood transfusion→ 'O' Negative should be given to patient

10. Antibody dependent killing:

a. NK cell
b. NK cell only
c. Macrophage
d. NK cell, neutrophils & macrophage

Ans. d. NK cell, neutrophils & macrophage

- ADCC—Antibody dependent cell mediated cytotoxicity is seen in NK cells, macrophages, neutrophils, eosinophils
- Phagocytosis
  - Opsonization/Recognization
  - Engulfment
  - Killing & degradation

11. Which of the following can recognize dead material?

a. NET
b. Inflammasome
c. Necrosis
d. Toll like receptor

Ans. d. Toll like receptor

- Clearance of necrotic cells is mediated by HMG β-1 receptor bounded by RAGE (receptor for advanced glycosylatoin end product) which is accepted by toll like receptor
- Toll like receptors are a class of proteins that play a key role in innate immune system. They are single, membrane spanning, non-catalytic receptors expressed on sentinel cells, such as macrophages, dendritic cells, natural killer cells, T and B lymphocytes, epithelial & endothelial cells and fibroblasts.
- Fraction

Upon activation (toll like receptors (TLRs) recruit adaptor proteins (proteins that mediate other protein - protein interaction)

↓

To propagate antigen induced signal transduction pathway

↓

Subsequent activation of protein kinase

↓

Reading to up regulation or suppression of genes that orchestrate inflammatory responses.

↓

If the binding ligand is bacteria

↓

Phagocytosis of bacteria is done and its antigens are presented to LD4 + T-cells.

↓

If ligand is viral factor—apoptosis of the veins infected cell

- Inflammasome multiprotein oligomer responsible for activation of inflammatory response like proinflammatory cytokines (IC-1, DC- 6, 8, TwF-α IwF-γ)

- Necrosis localised area of death of tissue followed latice by degradation of tissue by hydrolytic enzymes liberated from dead cells, invariably accompanied by inflammatory reaction.
- NET—(Neuroendocrine Tumor))

12. Immune privilege site is:

a. Optic nerve
b. Semi-inferous tubule
c. Area postern
d. Spinal cord

Ans. b. Semi-inferous tubule

- These are sites of human body which have ability to tolerate introduction of antigens without eliciting an inflammatory immune response. Tissue grafts not rejected in these sites.
- Include eyes
  - Placenta & fetus
  - Testicles
  - CNS

13. Immunofluorescene staining pattern from a kidney biopsy from a 35-year-old patient presenting with proteinuria has been shown below. What is the most probable cause?

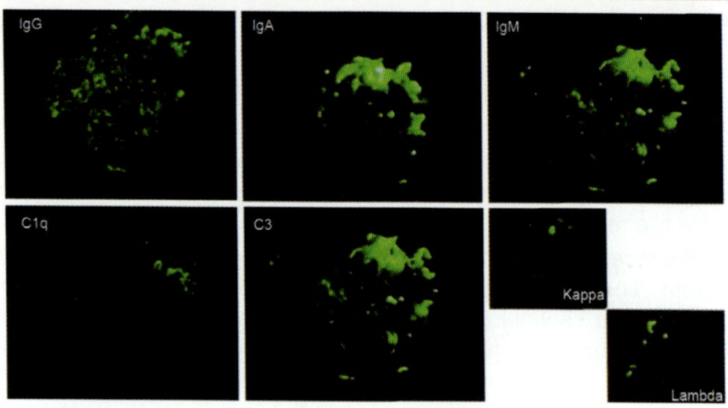

a. FSGS
b. PSGN
c. Lupus Nephritis
d. Goodpastures syndrome

Ans. c. Lupus nephritis

- We can see strong staining in IgA, IgM, C3 and weaker positive staining in IgG. Hence all are positive IgA, Ig M, C3, IgG commonly seen in SLE. as in SLE all types of glomerulonephritis seen.
- In FSGS→IgM & C3 (seen)
- In PSGN→IgG & C3 (seen)
- In Good pasture syndrome—IgG & C3 (seen) anti GBM disease

14. An intern while collecting blood split it over the floor. What should be done next?

a. Mop the floor
b. Put some absorbable material over it
c. 1% sodium hypochlorite
d. Inform the infection control board of hospital

Ans. b. Put some absorbable material over it

Protocol of a Blood spill

- Put protective clothes/gloves/apron
- Place a paper towel or absorbent material over the blood, cover it completely
- Clean the area with warm detergent solution, using disposable cloth or sponge
- You may use bleaching agents after cleaning

15. Anti-centromere antibodies seen in which of the followings conditions?

a. Drug induced lupus
b. SLE
c. Sjögren syndrome
d. Scleroderma

Ans. d. Scleroderma

Anticentromere antibodies are specific to centromere and kinetochore function occuring and syndactyly in (CREST syndrome).

C: Calcinosis
R: Raynaud's phenomenon
E: Esophageal dysmotility
S: Systemic scleroderma/sclerosis
T: Telangiectasia and syndactyly

16. Identify the marked structure in given below image:

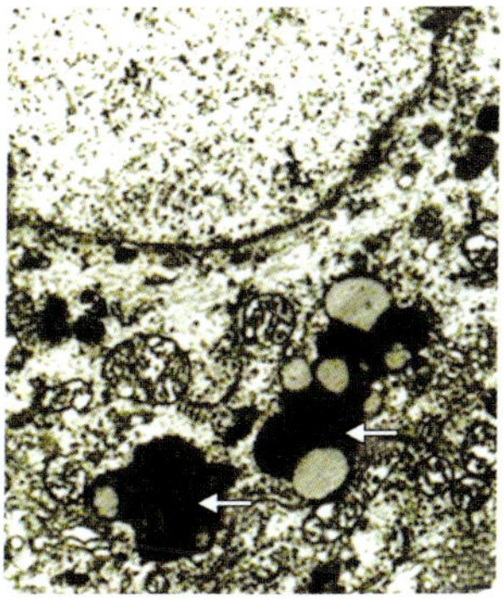

a. Lipofuscin granules
b. Lysosomes
c. Secondary lysosomes
d. Phagolysosome

Ans. a. Lipofuscin granules

- The marking area is the accumulation of lipofuscin granules
- It is also known as wear and tear pigment/Aging pigments
- It is telltale sign of free radical injury and lipid peroxidation
- It is perinuclear brown pigment
- It is seen in aging, severe malnutrition and cancer cachexia.

Primary lysosomes vs secondary lysosomes	
Primary lysosomes are membrane-bounded organelles that bud from the Golgi apparatus and contain many enzymes.	Secondary lysosomes are the organelles which form the combination of a primary lysosome and a phagosome or pinosome and in which lysis takes place through the activity of hydrolytic enzymes.

Contd...

Contd...

Formation	
Primary lysosomes are formed by the Golgi apparatus or ER complex.	Secondary lysosomes are formed by the fusion of primary lysosome with a phagosome or a pinosome.
Function	
Primary lysosomes are storage vacuoles.	Secondary lysosomes are digestive vacuoles.
Location	
Primary lysosomes are found in rough endoplasmic reticulum (RER).	Secondary lysosomes are found in the smooth endoplasmic reticulum (SER).
Exocytosis	
Primary lysosomes do not release its content.	Secondary lysosomes release its content outside into cytoplasm (exocytosis).
Biosynthesis	
Primary lysosomes do not involve in the biosynthesis in the useful materials to the cell.	Secondary lysosomes involved in the biosynthesis are important materials to the cell.
Acid hydrolases	
Waste products	Secondary lysosomes contain active acid hydrolases.
Primary lysosomes do not release waste products.	Secondary lysosomes release waste products through exocytosis.

PHARMACOLOGY

1. Dose reduction is required in renal failure with all *except*:

a. Amphotericin B
b. Vancomycin
c. Doxycycline
d. Gentamicin

Ans. c. Doxycycline

- Doxycycline is excreted mainly in feces through biliary excretion. No dose reduction required.
- For the rest dose reduction is required in renal failure
- Vancomycin may be associated with AKI.
- Aminoglycosides are freely filtered across the glomerulus and then accumulate within the renal cortex, where concentrations can greatly exceed those of the plasma.
- Amphotericin B causes renal vasoconstriction from an increase in tubulo-glomerular feedback as well as direct tubular toxicity mediated by reactive oxygen species. Nephrotoxicity from amphotericin B is dose and duration dependent.

2. Side effects of salbutamol are all *except*:

a. Hypokalemia
b. Hypoglycemia
c. Tremor
d. Tachycardia

Ans. b. Hypoglycemia

- The most common side effects of salbutamol are:
  - Muscle tremors
  - Tachycardia
  - Palpitation
  - Restlessness
  - Nervousness
  - Throat irritation
  - Ankle edema
  - Hypokalemia is a possible complication.

3. Loading dose depends on:

a. Volume of distribution
b. Bioavailability
c. Half-life
d. Clearance

Ans. a. Volume of distribution

- The loading dose is calculated as :
  - Loading dose = Css × Vd
    (Vd volume of distribution, Css steady state plasma concentration)
- Other important relationships:
  - Vd = dose / Cp
  - Maintinans dose = Cl × Css × dosing interval
  - Loading dose = Maintenance dose × 1.44 × t½

4. Low apparent volume of distribution indicates:

a. Drug is not extensively distributed in organs and tissues
b. Low bioavailability
c. Low T 1/2
d. Very low efficacy

Ans. a. Drug is not extensively distributed in organs and tissues

- Low apparent volume of distribution implies that the drug is restricted mainly to the intravascular compartment, and has low affinity for the target organs and tissues.
- *Volume of distribution* = $\frac{\text{Dose administered}}{\text{Plasma concentration}}$
- Plasma concentration will be high as drug is only in vascular compartment.

5. Pediatrician attended infant with unconjugated serum billrubin level of 33 mg/dL. Which drug mother might have taken in 3rd trimester?

a. Azithromycin
b. Chloroquine
c. Ampicillin
d. Cotrimoxazole

Ans. d. Cotrimoxazole

- Cotrimoxazole if given near term may cause Neonatal Hemolysis and Methemoglobinemia.
- Trimethoprim being an antifolate, there is theoretical teratogenic risk.
- Rest all the drugs are safe to be used during pregnancy.

6. For a patient of hypertension on metoprolol, verapamil was given; this will result in:

a. Atrial fibrillation
b. Bradycardia with AV block
c. Torsades de pointes
d. Tachycardia

Ans. b. Bradycardia with AV block

- Both beta blockers and verapamil have negative inotropic action which may be additive. Thus combining the two drugs cause decrease in heart rate and may also lead to AV block and prolongation of PR interval.

7. Mechanism by which Ach decreases heart rate is by?

a. Delayed diastolic depolarization
b. Increase in plateau
c. Decrease preload
d. Increase afterload

Ans. a. Delayed diastolic depolarization

- In the SA node, each normal cardiac impulse is initiated by the spontaneous depolarization of the pacemaker cells. Ach slows the heart rate primarily by decreasing the rate of spontaneous depolarization; attainment of the threshold potential and the succeeding events in the cardiac cycle are therefore delayed.

8. Diamox is given for glaucoma, which is a non-competitive antagonist of carbonic anhydrase. The effect is:

a. Increase in K_m and V_{max}
b. Decrease in K_m
c. Decrease in V_{max}
d. No change in V_{max}

Ans. c. Decrease in V_{max}

- *Noncompetitive antagonism*: Lowers V_{max} only
- *Uncompetitive antagonism*: Lowers both V_{max} and K_m
- *Competitive antagonism*: Raises K_m only

9. Which is gametocidal for all species?

a. Quinine
b. Chloroquine
c. Primaquine
d. None

Ans. c. Primaquine

- Primaquine is gametocidal to all species of Plasmodia while artemisinins have weak lethal action on early-stage but not mature gametes.
- Single 45 mg (0.75 mg/kg) dose of primaquine is employed immediately after clinical cure of falciparum malaria to kill the gametes and cut down transmission to mosquito.
- Quinine acts against asexual erythrocytic forms and has no significant effect on hepatic forms of malarial parasites.
- Chloroquine is highly effective against the erythrocytic forms of Plasmodia.

10. A male with insulin dependent diabetes having macular edema develops glaucoma. Which drug should be used as the least resort to treat?

a. Alpha agonist
b. Prostaglandin analogue
c. Pilocarpine
d. Beta blocker

Ans. c. Pilocarpine

- Pilocarpine is now used as a last resort for open angle glaucoma because it has several drawbacks—causes diminution of vision in dim light and patients with cataract, induces myopia, causes headache due to persistent spasm of iris and ciliary muscles, and also causes fluctuations in intraocular tension.

11. Lithium use in pregnancy leads to which effect on baby?

a. CVS defect
b. Urogenital defect
c. Neural tube defect
d. Facial defects

Ans. a. CVS defect

- Lithium is contraindicated during pregnancy. Fetal goiter and other congenital anomalies especially cardiac can occur. The newborn is often hypotonic.
- Lithium is associated with Ebstein's anomaly.

12. If carbamazepine is added to valproate, which of the following side-effect increases?

a. Thrombocytopenia
b. Hepatotoxicity
c. Hyperammonemia
d. Pancreatitis

Ans. b. Hepatotoxicity

- Asymptomatic rise in serum transaminase is often noted in valproate; and monitoring of liver function is advised. Those with hepatic disease or who receive other anticonvulsant/hepatotoxic drug (e.g. carbamazepine) are at greater risk to develop fulminant hepatitis.

13. Which of the following drug is used to prevent acute mountain sickness?

a. Acetazolamide
b. Dexamethasone
c. Diltiazem
d. Digoxin

Ans. a. Acetazolamide

- Acetazolamide is used for symptomatic relief as well as prophylaxis in acute mountain sickness. Benefit occurs probably due to reduced CSF formation as well as lowering of CSF and brain pH.
- MOA:
  - at high altitude respiratory rate will increases which causes respiratory alkalosis.
  - Acetazolamide causes metabolic acidosis by following mechanism.

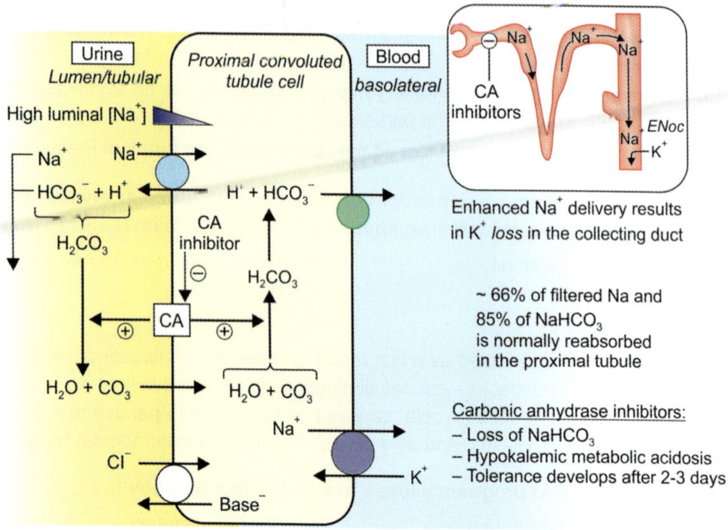

14. A known case of TB is now resistant to Rifampicin and Isoniazid. Which of the following would be most appropriate in treating this patient?

a. 6 drugs for 4 months; 4 drugs for 12 months
b. 6 drugs for 6 months; 4 drugs for 18 months
c. 4 drugs for 4 months, 6 drugs for 12 months
d. 5 drugs for 2 months; 4 drugs for 1 months; 3 drugs for 5 months

Ans. b. 6 drugs for 6 months; 4 drugs for 18 months.

The general principle of treatment of MDR-TB are:

- At least 4 drugs certain to be effective. Often 5–6 drugs are included since efficacy of some are uncertain
- Avoid combining cross-resistant drugs e.g. two FQs, Kanamycin with Amikacin or Ethionamide with Pyrazinamide or Cycloserine with terizidone
- Include drugs from group 1 to group IV in a hierarchical order. Group I drugs (except H and R can be included, add one injectable drug (Group II) and one or two Group IV drugs
- RNTCP has devised a 'standardized' treatment regimen of 6 drugs intensive phase lasting 6-9 months and 4 continuation phase of 18 months.

15. Schedule of drug to be sold only on prescription is:

a. H
b. P
c. G
d. X

Ans. a. H

Important Drug Schedules in India

Schedule G	List of drugs that do not need prescription but requires a mandatory text on lable " Caution: It is dangerous to take this preparation, except under medical supervision, e.g. antihistaminics
Schedule H	List of drugs that can be sold only when a prescription is produced. Most drugs belong to this category
Schedule P	It is about drug expiry period i.e. maximum period till which drug can be use with intact potency
Schedule W	List of drugs marketed under generic names only
Schedule X	List of psychotropic drugs which need special license for manufactures and sale
Schedule Y	Guidelines on clinical trials, import and manufacture of new drugs

16. In a rheumatic heart disease pregnant female with prosthetic valve, when should we switch to heparin?

a. 32 weeks
b. 36 weeks
c. 37 weeks
d. 40 weeks

Ans. b. 36 weeks

The European Society of Cardiology as well as the ACC/AHA recommends:

Heparin during the 1st trimester (to avoid warfarin embryopathy), followed by oral anticoagulation up to the 36th week with subsequent replacement by heparin until delivery.

17. Phase 1 trial is done to test:

a. Safety
b. Efficacy
c. Dose
d. Pharmacokinetics

Ans. a. Safety

- *Preclinical*: Non-human subjects, to gather efficacy, toxicity and pharmacokinetic information
- *Phase 0*: Microdose Pharmacokinetics
- *Phase I*: Safety, tolerability, and to detect any potentially dangerous effects on vital functions.
- *Phase II*: Therapeutic efficacy, dose range and ceiling effect in a controlled setting. Tolerability and pharmacokinetics as an extension of Phase I
- *Phase III*: Safety and tolerability, establish value of drug in relation to existing therapy.
- *Phase IV*: Uncommon/idiosyncratic adverse effects

18. Nitroprusside active metabolite act by:

a. Phosphokinase 1.2
b. Guanylyl cyclase
c. Phospholipase A
d. Phospholipase B

Ans. b. Guanylyl cyclase

- Nitroprusside is a light-sensitive, short-acting agent (duration of action is a few minutes) that must be infused continuously. The release of Nitric Oxide from the drug molecule itself stimulates guanylyl cyclase and increases cyclic guanine monophosphate (cGMP) concentration and relaxation in vascular smooth muscle.

19. Dapsone is used as antibacterial, antifungal and as immunomodulator. What is the mechanism behind all these actions?

a. Inhibition of cell wall synthesis
b. Inhibition of sterol of the cell wall
c. Inhibition of protein synthesis in ribosomes
d. Competes with PABA in folic acid synthesis

Ans. d. Competes with PABA in folic acid synthesis

Dapsone is a competitive antagonist of para-aminobenzoic acid (PABA) and prevents normal bacterial utilization of PABA for the synthesis of folic acid.

20. The kit in the picture is used for treatment of:

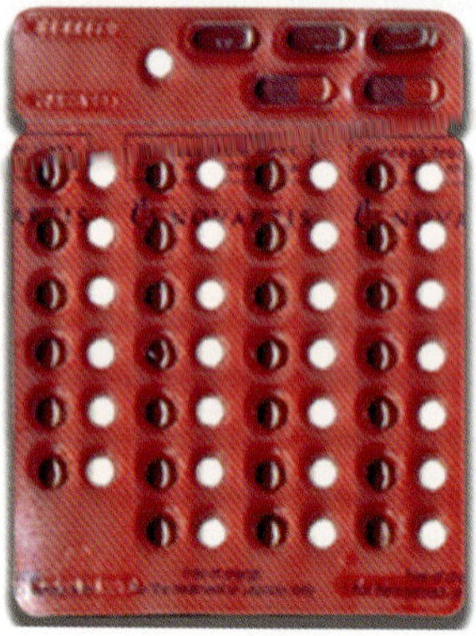

a. HIV
b. Leprosy
c. Urethral discharge
d. TB

Ans. b. Leprosy

- *Multibacillary leprosy*: (WHO) Dapsone (100 mg/day) plus Clofazimine (50 mg/day) unsupervised and Rifampin (600 mg) plus clofazimine (300 mg) monthly supervised for 1-2 years
- *Paucibacillary leprosy*: (WHO) Dapsone (100 mg/day) unsupervised plus rifampin (600 mg) plus clofazimine (300 mg) monthly supervised for 6 months.

21. Morphine should not be given in a patient with:

a. Ischemic pain
b. Cancer pain
c. Biliary colic
d. Postoperative pain

Ans. c. Biliary colic

- Opioids contract biliary smooth muscle, which can result in biliary colic. The sphincter of Oddi may constrict, resulting in reflux of biliary and pancreatic secretions and elevated plasma amylase and lipase levels.

22. A patient is on indinavir, zidovudine, lamivudine and ketoconazole. He developed breast hypertrophy, nephrolithiasis, hyperlipidemia and central obesity; identify the drug causing these side effects amongst all:

a. Lamivudine
b. Indinavir
c. Ketoconazole
d. Zidovudine

Ans. b. Indinavir

- The most common side effects of indinavir are—GI disturbances, malaise, fatigue, nephrolithiasis/urolithiasis, metabolic alterations-hyperlipidemia, hyperglycemia, lipodystrophy (Crix belly), hyperbilirubinemia, renal abnormalities etc.
- Lamivudine—well tolerated. Lipoatrophy in some cases
- Ketoconazole—GI disturbances, itching, headache, dizziness, impotence, decreased libido
- Zidovudine—Anemia, neutropenia, lipoatrophy

23. Which of the following is correct regarding T3 and T4 acting on TRH?

a. It activates phospholipase A
b. It acts on transcription factor
c. It acts by increasing cAMP
d. It is a tyrosine kinase receptor

Ans. b. It acts on transcription factor

- Increased thyroid hormone inhibits transcription of both the TRH gene and the genes encoding the α .and β subunits of TSH, which suppresses the secretion of TSH and causes the thyroid to become inactive and regress.

24. A 16-year-old girl was on antiepileptic for treatment of seizure episodes while asleep. She had no seizure for 6 months and NCCT and EEG was normal. What is further management?

a. Stop treatment
b. Continue for 2 years
c. Lifelong treatment
d. Stop treatment and follow up with 6 monthly EEG

Ans. b. Continue for 2 years

- Once initiated, Anti-seizure drugs are typically continued for 2 years. Tapering and discontinuing therapy should be considered if the patient is seizure free after 2 years; tapering should be done slowly over several months. Typically, 80% of recurrences will occur within 4 months of discontinuing therapy.

25. Antitubercular drug causing ophthalmic toxicity is:

a. Isoniazid
b. Rifampicin
c. Ethambutol
d. None of above

Ans. c. Ethambutol

- *Ethambutol*: Optic neuritis, resulting in decreased visual acuity and loss of red-green discrimination. Other side effects—pruritus, joint pain, GI upset, abdominal pain, malaise, headache, dizziness, mental confusion, disorientation, and possible hallucinations. Increased concentration of urate in blood.
- *Isoniazid:* Hepatotoxicity (elevated serum aspartate, alanine transaminases), peripheral neuritis (pyridoxine to be given concurrently), convulsions, optic neuritis, atrophy, muscle twitching, dizziness, ataxia, paresthesias, stupor, toxic encephalopathy. Euphoria, transient impairment of memory loss of self-control, and florid psychosis may occur. Hypersensitivity, hematological reactions, arthritis, dryness of mouth, epigastric distress, methemoglobinemia, tinnitus, urinary retention, anemia, SLE may also occur.
- *Rifampicin*: Rash, flu-like fever, chills, myalgias nausea and vomiting. Rarely hepatitis. Hypersenstitivity, eosinophilia, interstitial nephritis, acute tubular necrosis, thrombocytopenia, hemolytic anemia, and shock. Light chain proteinuria has also been documented. Potential teratogenic.

26. All of the following drugs increase bleeding when given to a patient on warfarin *except:*

a. Isoniazid
b. Amiodarone
c. Carbamazepine
d. Cimetidine

Ans. c. Carbamazepine

- Amiodarone, Cimetidine, Isoniazid inhibit warfarin metabolism (CYP2C9), thus increased serum concentrations of warfarin, leading to bleeding symptoms.
- Carbamazepine on the other hand causes increase in warfarin metabolism (through CYP2C9 induction), thus decreasing the serum concentration of Warfarin and does not cause bleeding. Increase in warfarin dose of 50–100% required when initiating CBZ.

Cytochrome P-450 interactions (selected)

Inducers (+)	Substrates	Inhibitors (–)
Chronic alcohol use	Anti-epileptics	Sodium valproate
St John's wort	Theophylline	Isoniazid
Phenytoin	Warfarin	Cimetidine
Phenobarbital	OCPs	Ketoconazole
Nevirapine		Fluconazole
Rifampin		Fluconazole
Griseofulvin		Acute alcohol abuse
Carbamazepine		Chloramphenicol
		Erythromycin (macrolides)
		Sulfonamides
		Ciprofloxacin
		Omeprazole
		Metronidazole

27. Primary action of nitrates in patient of angina is:

a. Coronary vasodilation
b. Decreases preload
c. Decreases afterload
d. Decreases heart rate

Ans. b. Decreases preload

- When GTN is directly injected into the coronary circulation of patients with CAD, anginal attacks are not aborted even when coronary blood flow is increased. However, sublingual administration of GTN does relieve angina pain in some, indicating that the major antianginal effect of nitrovasodilators is mediated by preload reduction rather than coronary artery dilation.
- Nitrovasodilators preferentially decrease preload by dilating venous capacitance vessels.
- The decrease in afterload is generally small and mainly observed at higher doses.
- NO and nitrovasodilators can directly modulate the inotropic or chronotropic state of the heart via cGMP and its stimulatory effect on PDE2 or an inhibitory effect on the cAMP-specific PDE3.

28. The technique given in the picture is used for:

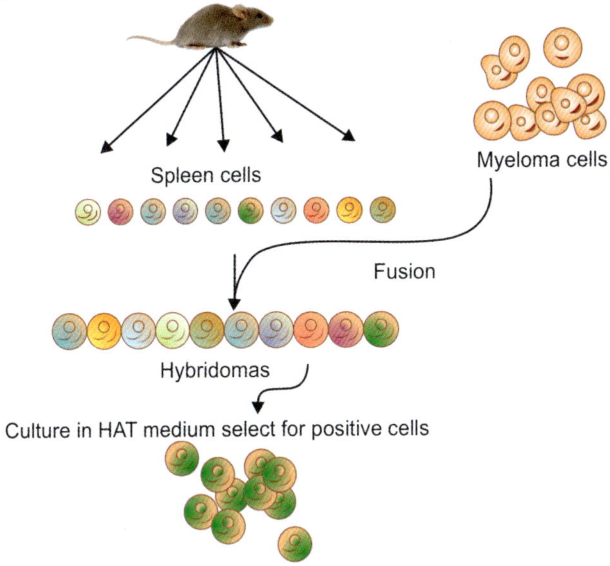

a. Synthesis of monoclonal antibodies
b. Preparing cell lines for viral culture
c. Synthesis of vaccine
d. Process of genetic engineering

Ans. a. Synthesis of monoclonal antibodies

- Hybridoma selection after fusion of myelomas and spleen cells is a critical step in monoclonal body production. HAT method is used to accomplish the task.
- Unfused spleen cells are easily selected against since they do not replicate in culture.
- Unfused myelomas can be selected against using media containing HAT (hypoxanthine-aminopterin-thymidine). The aminopterin found in the medium blocks the de novo DNA nucleotide synthesis pathway. Typically when the de novo pathway is blocked, cells will then utilize the salvage pathway as an alternative means to replicate (only if hypoxanthine and thymidine are present). However, these myelomas are unable to do so since they are deficiont in an enzyme called HGPRT, which is required for the salvage pathway. Hence, myelomas are unable to replicate in culture.

Only hybridomas survive. Hybridomas inherit a functioning HGPRT enzyme from the spleen cells, so even though the de novo pathway is blocked, they can still use the salvage pathway to replicate.

29. Store a drug in a cool place refers to:

a. Below freezing point of water
b. 0°
c. 2°–4°
d. 8°–15°

Ans. d. 8°–15°

- Storing frozen: –20°C
- Storing at cool temperature: 8°–15°C
- Storing at ambient temperature: 15°–25°C

MICROBIOLOGY

1. 200 people attended a party and some of them had diarrhea after 24 hours. They ate oyster, hamburger, icecream and potato salad. What is the likely cause?

40 ill from 50 who consumed oyster

50 ill from 135 who consumed hamburger

60 ill from 140 who consumed salad

49 ill from 115 who consumed icecream

a. V. parahaemolyticus
b. Salmonella enteritidis
c. Yersinia enterocolitis
d. Staph aureus

Ans. a. V. parahaemolyticus.

- Incidence of diarrhea is maximum in oyster eating population.
- It is most likely causative agent, it is found in raw oyster from contaminated oyster beds, usually in late summer. Associated with mild gastroenteritis. Also found in raw fish and sushi.
- Why not.....
  - Salmonella enteritidis is more commonly transmitted through infected eggs. Consumption of undercooked eggs is major risk factor. It can cause diarrhea within 12–72 hour after consumption of infected food.
  - Yersinia enterocolitis causes acute diarrhea, terminal ileitis and mesenteric lymphadenitis and pseudoappendicitis. Human yersiniosis is attributed to contaminated PORK, MILK, WATER and TOFU.
  - Staphylococcal food poisoning results from the ingestion of preformed enterotoxins, which have rapid onset of (1 to 6 hours) nausea and vomiting and usually resolve in less than 24 hours without treatment.
- Incidence of diarrhea in oyster eating population is more

2. A patient is having thick, gray coating on the throat and tonsils, followed with fever, chills and swollen glands in the week. Microscopic examination of nasopharyngeal or pharyngeal swab showed gram positive organism with a special stain. The constitutes of the stain are:

a. Crystal violet, Gram's iodine
b. Toluidine blue, malachite green, glacial acetic
c. Carbol fuchsin, acid alcohol, and methylene blue
d. Methylene blue

Ans. b. Toluidine blue, malachite green, glacial acetic

- Clinical features in question is pointing towards diphtheria. Albert stain is used to stain metachromatic granules of Corynebacterium diphtheriae.
- Albert stain is made up of two stains Toluidine blue O, malachite green and glacial acetic acid.
- Toluidine blue O stains volutin granules (most acidic part of cell) and Malachite green stains cytoplasm blue green.

Why not.....

- ❑ Option A is grams stain, easily rule out because not special stain for C. diphtheriae
- ❑ Option C is Modified ZN stain.
- ❑ Methylene blue is cationic stain binds to negatively charge parts of cells such as nucleic acids DNA in nucleus and RNA in cytoplasm (with lower affinity). Methylene blue is agent of choice for staining pus cells.

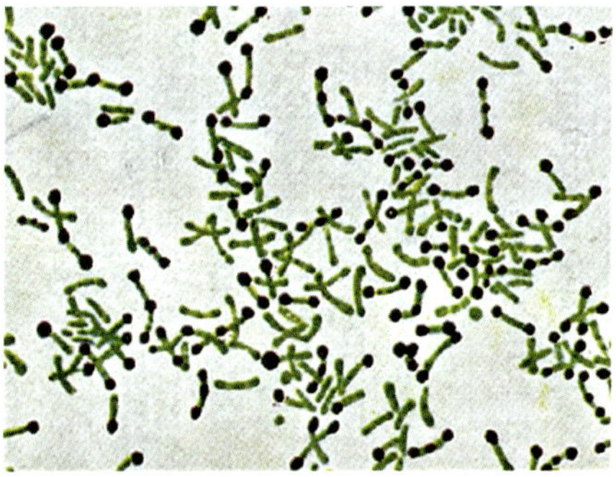

Albert stain of diphtheria

3. Postrenal transplant patient presents with diarrhea after 3 months; it was showing organism measuring 2–6 micron meter and kinyoun stain positive. Most likely it is caused by:

a. Balantidium coli b. Clostridium difficile
c. Cystoisospora belli d. Cryptosporidium hominis

Ans d. cryptosporidium hominis

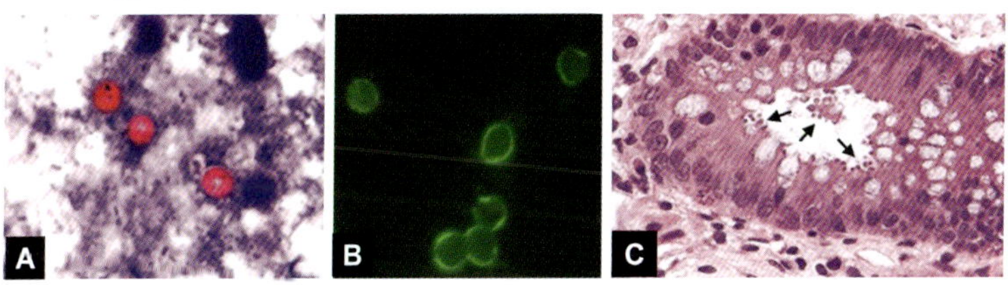

Cryptosporidium (A) acid fast; (B) fluorescent, (C) intestinal histopathology (see arrow)

- ❑ It causes diarrhea in immunocompromised patients.
  - ❍ Clinically present as abdominal pain and cramps, watery diarrhea.

Lab Dx:

- ❑ Direct microscopy (stool examination) shows round 4–6 micrometer size oocyst: Cysts in acid fast stain of stool.
- ❑ Antigen detection from stool: ICT and ELISA
- ❑ Antibody detection from serum: ELISA
- ❑ Molecular diagnosis: PCR
- ❑ Histopathology of intestinal biopsy specimen.
- ❑ Nitazoxanide for severe diarrhea. Cause of large community-wide outbreaks from contaminated water supply
- ❑ Acid fast stain include Z-N stain, Kinyoun stain, fite stain.

- Fite stain is used for Nocardia.
- Kinyoun stain is used for staining of mycobacteria, cryptosporidium species, C. belli and cyclospora cayetanensis.

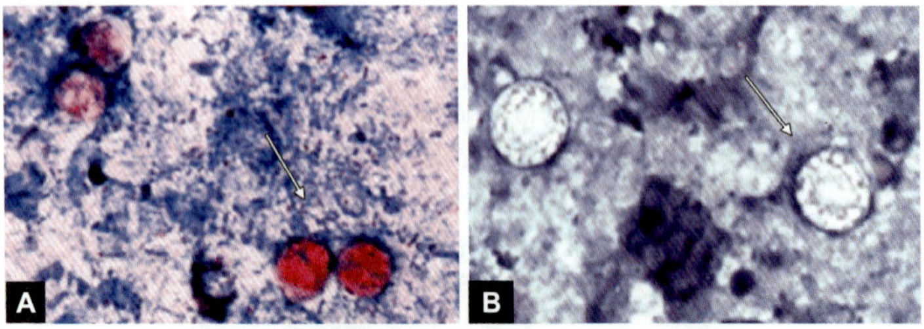

- Acid fast stain of cyclospara
- *Balantidium coli* trophozoites and cysts are found in stool.
- Trophozoites are large size 40–200 micrometer and cysts are 50–70 micrometer in size. *B coli* can also invade tissue.
- *B. coli* is the largest protozoan and only ciliate parasite that infect humans.

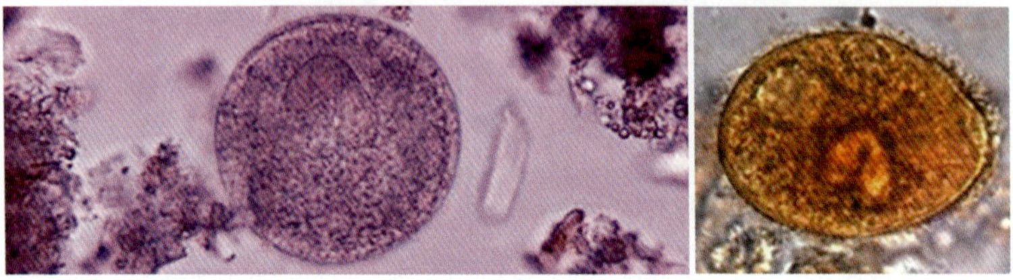

Balantidium coli

Property	Cryptosporidium	Cyclospora	Isospora
Infective form	Sporulated oocyst	Sporulated oocyst	Sporulated oocyst
Diagnostic form	Sporulated oocyst	Unsporulated oocyst	Unsporulated oocyst
Outbreakes	Common	Occasional	Occasional
Oocyst size	4–6 µm	8–10 µm	23–36 µm
Oocyst shape	Round	Round	Oval
Sporulated oocyst contain	Four sporozoites	Two sporoblast, each having two sporozoites	Two sporoblast, each having four sporozoites
Acid fastness	Uniformly acid fast	Variable acid fast	Uniformly acid fast
Autofluorescence	No, but can be stained with fluorescent dye	Autofluorescence ++	Autofluorescence +/–
Sporulation of the oocyst	Occurs inside the host cells (enterocytes)	Occurs in soil (environment)	Occurs in soil (environment)
Treatment	Nitazoxanide	Cotrimoxazole	Cotrimoxazole

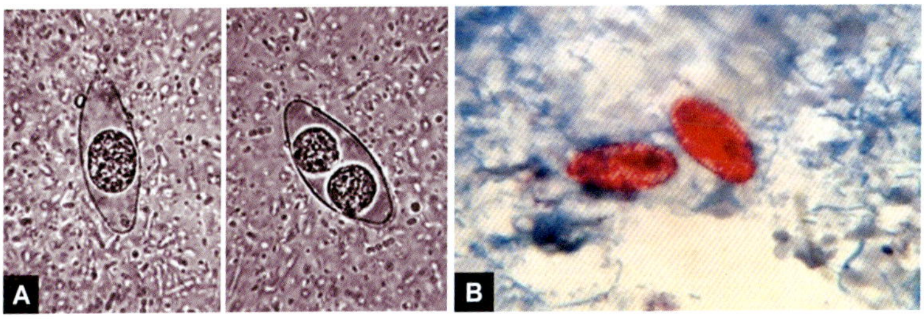

Isospora belli (A) saline mount preparation shows left—unsporulated occyst and right—sporulated oocyst; (B) modified acid fast stain shows unsporulated oocyst

4. Small amounts of repeated thin stools with mucus, subjective feeling of fever and lower abdominal pain, with leukocytes in stool. Which of the following is likely?

a. Giardia
b. Entamoeba
c. Staph
d. Clostridium perfringens

Ans. b. Entamoeba

- Since diarrhea is inflammatory type a/w leukocytes in stool and fever (large bowel).
- Why not clostridium perfringes? Because no recent antibiotics use history.
- Approach to diarrhea in adults:
  - Diarrhea from small bowel typically watery, large volume and associated with abdominal cramping, bloating and gas. Weight loss can occur if diarrhea is persistent, fever is rarely significant and occult blood in stool and inflammatory cells in stool are rarely identified.
  - Diarrhea from large bowel presents with frequent, regular, small volume and often painful bowel movements. Fever and bloody or mucoid stools are common and red blood cells and inflammatory can be seen routinely on stool microscopy.

Pathogen	Small bowel	Colon
Bacteria	❑ *Salmonella* ❑ *Escherichia coli* ❑ *Clostridium perfringens* ❑ *Staphylococcus aureus* ❑ *Aeromonas hydrophila* ❑ *Bacillus cereus* ❑ *Vibrio cholerae*	❑ *Campylobacter* ❑ *Shigella* ❑ *Clostridioides difficile* ❑ *Yersinia* ❑ *Vibrio parahaemolyticus* ❑ *Enteroinvasive E. coli* ❑ *Plesiomonas shigelloides* ❑ *Klebsiella oxytoca (rare)*
Virus	❑ Rotavirus ❑ Norovirus ❑ Astrovirus	❑ Cytomegalovirus ❑ Adenovirus ❑ Herpes simplex virus
Protozoa	❑ Cryptosporidium ❑ Microsporidium ❑ Cystoisospora ❑ Cyclospora ❑ Giardia lamblia	❑ Entamoeba histolytica

5. IFN beta stimulated by:

a. Bacterial infection
b. Viral infection
c. Fungal infection
d. Mycoplasma infection

Ans. b. Viral infected

- IFN can modulate lymphocyte function either directly (e.g. in case of natural killer cell activity) or indirectly through modulation of major histocompatibility complex.
- Antiviral effects by induction or activation of several enzyme systems which prevents synthesis of viral protein.
- IFN activates NK cells activity. IFN $\alpha\beta$ can up regulate class I MHC antigens but not class II while IFN Υ can upregulate both MHC I and II (MCH II on certain cell types e.g. macrophages).
- MOA: Cells activated to produce IFNs secrete it into extracellular space then it diffuses to other cells, binds to specific receptor (single receptor for $\alpha\beta$ and separate for Υ) Subsequent to this binding a number of genes activated resulting in protein production responsible for action of IFNs.
- IFN α, IFN β are secreted by viral infected cells.
- IFN Υ is produced by T lymphocytes, T_H and T_C cells, NK cells upon mitogenic stimulus. It activates resting macrophages into activated macrophages. It activates B cells to produce IgG. Along with TNF β promotes inflammation of delayed types of hypersensitivity. Inhibits T_H2 cell proliferation.

6. Patient with history of Kidney transplantation presenting with diarrhea. (Video of worms given). The motility of the worms given in the figure. Correct statement about the organism is:

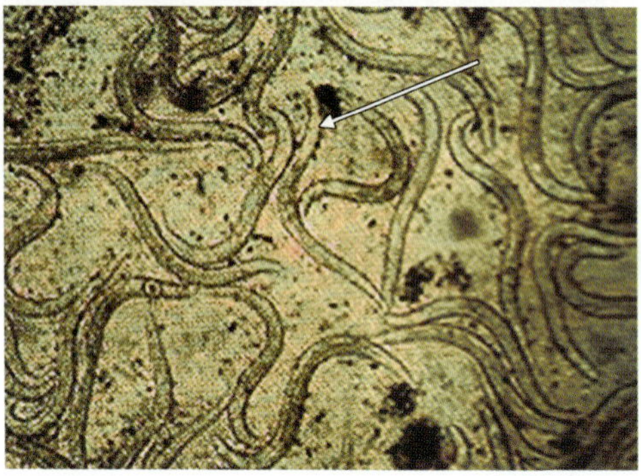

a. Monoecious and the organism related with parthenogenesis.
b. Transmitted by intake contaminated food and water
c. Loffler's pneumonia is not caused by the same organism.
d. Body gets this infection through filariform larvae.

Ans. d. Body gets this infection through filariform larvae.

- Larvae in stool classically seen in *Strongyloides stercoralis.*

Why not

- *Strongyloides stercoralis* is *dioicous, male and female both forms exist.*
- Mode of transmission is skin penetration by filariform larvae.
- Larvae migrate via the bloodstream to the lungs, where they are eventually coughed up and swallowed. *Strongyloides stercoralis causes Loffler's pneumonia.*

Parthenogenesis: Compared with most other parasitic nematodes, the *Strongyloides* life cycle is unusual because it has two adult generations – one in the host and one outside The parasitic adult generation is female-only and these reproduce by parthenogenesis, which is genetically mitotic The parasitic females produce eggs that are, genetically, male and female. These eggs, or the L1s that hatch from the eggs, pass out of the host in its feces (which stage is passed being a species-specific character), where the larvae then grow, develop and moult. Males and females have different developmental fates. Male eggs (or larvae) moult through four larval stages (L1–L4) and then into free-living adult male worms. The female eggs (or larvae) have a developmental choice. In one option, they can develop analogously to males (moulting through four larval stages) finally moulting into free-living adult female worms. Alternatively the female larvae can moult through three larval stages into third-stage larvae (L3s), which are infectious to a new host.

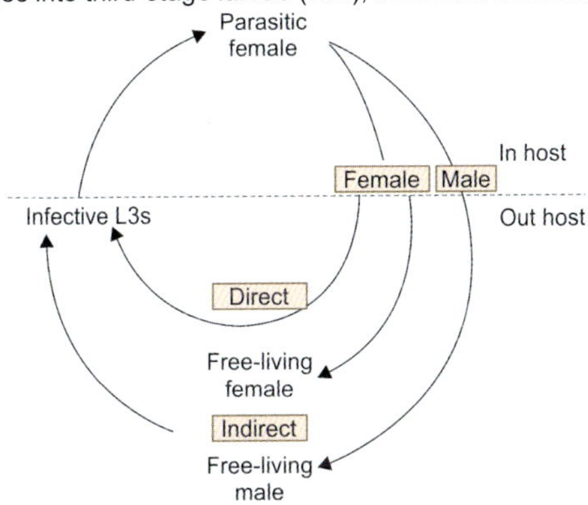

Life cycle of *Strongyloides stercoralis.*

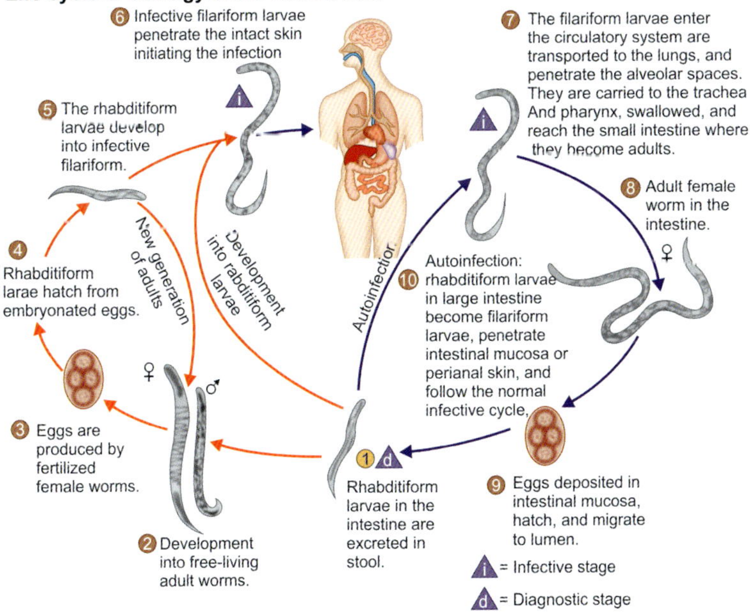

7. TB is transmitted through droplets mode of transmission; which other disease also has droplet mode of transmission and isolation is done:

a. Pertussis
b. Atypical pneumonia
c. Faucial diphtheria
d. Hepatitis B

Ans. a. Pertussis

- Both diphtheria and pertussis can be transmitted by droplet infection but isolation required in pertussis. In pertussis isolation in a quite environment may inhibits the stimulation of paroxysms.

Types of Precautions for Infection Control

Type of precaution	Selected patients	Major specifications
Standard	All patients	❑ Perform hand hygiene before and after every patient contact. ❑ Gloves, gowns, eye protection as required. ❑ Safe disposal or cleaning of instruments and linen. ❑ Cough etiquette: Patients and visitors should cover their nose or mouth when coughing, promptly dispose used tissues, and practice hand hygiene after contact with respiratory secretions.
Contact	❑ Colonization of any bodily site with multi-drug-resistant bacteria (MRSA, VRE, drug-resistant gram-negative organisms) ❑ Enteric infections (Norovirus, *Clostridioides* (formerly *Clostridium*) *difficile*, *Escherichia coli* O157:H7) ❑ Viral infections (HSV, VZV, RSV, parainfluenza, enterovirus, rhinovirus) ❑ Scabies ❑ Impetigo ❑ Noncontained abscesses or decubitus ulcers (especially for *Staphylococcus aureus* and group A *Streptococcus*)	In addition to standard precautions: ❑ Private room preferred; cohorting allowed if necessary. ❑ Gloves required upon entering room. Change gloves after contact with contaminated secretions. ❑ Gown required if clothing may come into contact with the patient or environmental surfaces or if the patient has diarrhea. ❑ Minimize risk of environmental contamination during patient transport (e.g. patient can be placed in a gown). ❑ Noncritical items should be dedicated to use for a single patient if possible.

Contd…

Contd…

Type of precaution	Selected patients	Major specifications
Droplet	Known or suspected: ❑ *Neisseria meningitidis* ❑ *Haemophilus influenzae* type B ❑ *Mycoplasma pneumoniae* ❑ *Bordetella pertussis* ❑ Group A *Streptococcus* ❑ Diphtheria ❑ Pneumonic plague ❑ Influenza ❑ Rubella ❑ Mumps ❑ Adenovlrus ❑ Parvovirus Bl9 ❑ Rhinovirus	In addition to standard precautions: ❑ Place the patient in an AIIR (a monitored negative pressure room with at least 6 to 12 air exchanges per hour). ❑ Room exhaust must be appropriately discharged outdoors or passed through a HEPA filter before recirculation within the hospital. ❑ A certified respirator must be worn when entering the room of a patient with diagnosed or suspected tuberculosis. ❑ Susceptible individuals should not enter the room of patients with confirmed or suspected measles or chickenpox. ❑ Transport of the patient should be minimized; the patient should be masked if transport within the hospital is unavoidable ❑ *Cough etiquette*: Patients and visitors should cover their nose or mouth when coughing, promptly dispose used tissues, and practice hand hygiene after contact with respiratory secretions.
Airborne	Known or suspected: ❑ Tuberculosis ❑ Varicella ❑ Measles ❑ Smallpox ❑ SARS ❑ Ebola	In addition to standard precautions: ❑ Place the patient in an AIIR (a monitored negative pressure room with at least 6 to 12 air exchanges per hour). ❑ Room exhaust must be appropriately discharged outdoors or passed through a HEPA filter before recirculation within the hospital. ❑ A certified respirator must be worn when entering the room of a patient with diagnosed or suspected tuberculosis. ❑ Susceptible individuals should not enter the room of patients with confirmed or suspected measles or chickenpox. ❑ Transport of the patient should be minimized; the patient should be masked if transport within the hospital is unavoidable. ❑ *Cough etiquette:* Patients and visitors should cover their nose or mouth when coughing, promptly dispose used tissues, and practice hand hygiene after contact with respiratory secretions.

8. Vaccines include in NIS all, *except*:

a. Rota virus
b. Influenza
c. Adult JE
d. Hep-B

Ans. a. Rota virus

- Rota virus is not included in NIS schedule.

National Immunization Schedule (NIS) for Infants, Children and Pregnant Women

Vaccine	When to give	Dose	Route	Site
For pregnant women				
TT-1	Early in pregnancy	0.5 mL	Intramuscular	Upper arm
TT-2	4 weeks after TT-1*	0.5 mL	Intramuscular	Upper arm
TT- Booster	If received 2 TT doses in pregnancy within the last 3 yrs	0.5 ml	Intramuscular	Upper arm
For infants				
BCG	At birth or as early as possible till one year of age	0.1 mL (0.05 mL until 1 month age)	Intradermal	Left upper arm
Hepatitis B – Birth dose	At birth or as early as possible within 24 hours	0.5 mL	Intramuscular	Antero-lateral side of mid-thigh
OPV-0	At birth or as early as possible within the first 15 days	2 drops	Oral	Oral
OPV 1, 2 & 3	At 6 weeks, 10 weeks and 14 weeks (OPV can be given till 5 years of age)	2 drops	Oral	Oral
Pentavalent 1, 2 & 3	At 6 weeks, 10 weeks and 14 weeks (can be given till one year of age)	0.5 mL	Intramuscular	Antero – lateral side of mid-thigh
Rotavirus#	At 6 weeks, 10 weeks and 14 weeks (can be given till one year of age)	5 drops	Oral	Oral
IPV	Two fractional dose at 6 and 14 weeks of age	0.1 mL	Intradermal two fractional dose	Intradermal: Right upper arm

Contd…

Contd…

Vaccine	When to give	Dose	Route	Site
Measles/MR 1st Dose$	9 completed months-12 months. (can be given till 5 years of age)	0.5 mL	Subcutaneous	Right upper arm
JE-1**	9 completed month-12 months.	0.5 mL	Subcutaneous	Left upper arm
Vitamin A (1st dose)	At 9 completed months with measles-Rubella	1 mL (1 lakh IU)	Oral	Oral
For children				
DPTbooster-1	16–24 months	0.5 mL	Intramuscular	Anterolateral side of mid-thigh
Measles/MR 2nd dose$	16–24 months	0.5 mL	Subcutaneous	Right upper arm
OPV Booster	16–24 months	2 drops	Oral	Oral
JE-2	16–24 months	0.5 mL	Subcutaneous	Left upper arm
Vitamin A* (2nd to 9th dose)**	16–18 months. Then one dose every 6 months up to the age of 5 years	2 mL (2 lakh IU)	Oral	Oral
DPT Booster-2	5–6 years	0.5 mL	Intramuscular	Upper arm
TT	10 years & 16 years	0.5 mL	Intramuscular	Upper arm

* Give TT-2 or Booster doses before 36 weeks of pregnancy. However, give these even if more than 36 weeks have passed. Give TT to a woman in labour, if she has not previously received TT.

* JE Vaccine is introduced in select endemic districts after the campaign.

***The 2nd to 9th doses of Vitamin A can be administered to children 1–5 years old during biannual rounds, in collaboration with ICDS.

\# Phased introduction, at present in Andhra Pradesh, Haryana, Himachal Pradesh and Orissa from 2016 & expanded in Madhya Pradesh, Assam, Rajasthan, and Tripura in February 2017 and planned in Tamil Nadu & Uttar Pradesh in 2017.

$ Phased introduction, at present in five states namely Karnataka, Tamil Nadu, Goa, Lakshadweep and Puducherry. (As of Feb' 2017)

9. The causative agent of Bacterial meningitis in a 1 year child:

a. Pneumococcus
b. H. influenza
c. Neisseria meningitides
d. Listeria

Ans. a. Pneumococcus

Most common cause of bacterial meningitis in infants is Pneumococcus.

Common causes of meningitis in infants.

Ist S pneumoniae
IInd N meningitis (Ist in teens)
IIIrd H influenzae type B
IVth Enteroviruses

Acute bacterial meningitis:

- *Up to 2 months*: Listeria monocytogenes
- *2-3 month*: Pneumococcus
- *3 month-2 year*: world pneumococcus India: H. influenzae
- *2-12 year*: pneumococcus

Ref: Jawetz's medical microbiology

10. Life cycle shown in figure is of:

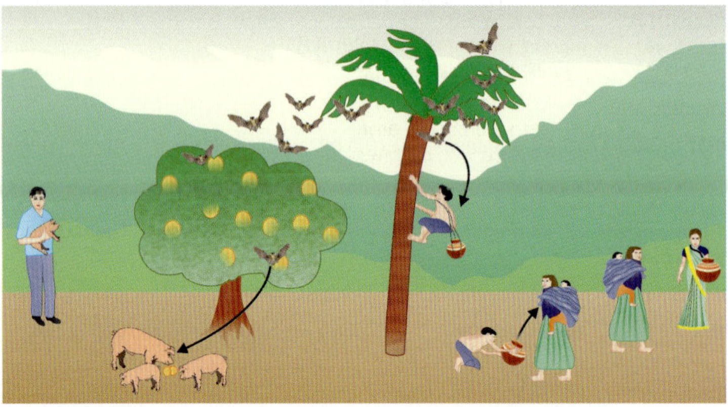

a. Nipah   b. Rabies virus
c. JE   d. West nile virus

Ans. a. Nipah

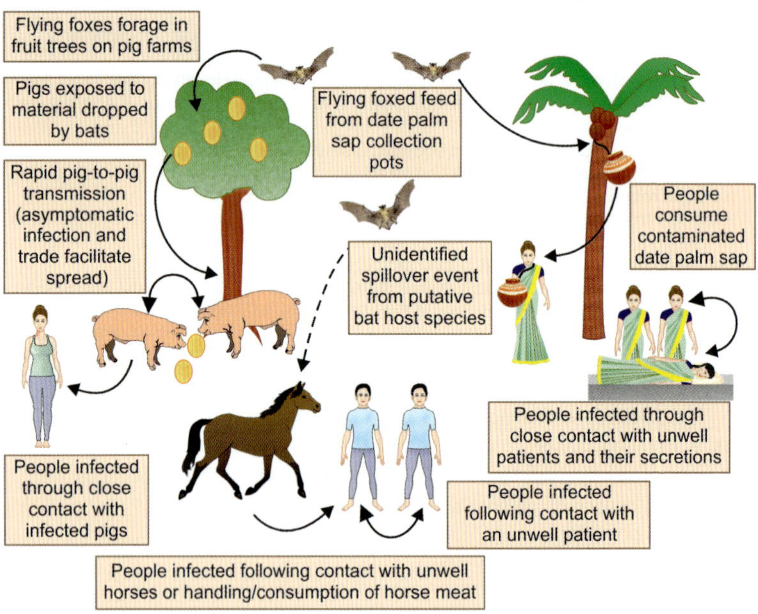

- As mentioned in picture bats are mode of transmission, which is not in case of JE and West nile.
- Nipah virus was initially isolated and identified in 1999 during an outbreak of encephalitis and respiratory illness among pig farmer and in people with close contact with pig in Malaysia and Singapore. Named NIPAH based on Malaysian village "sungai nipah".
- Transmission: infected bats and infected pigs
- Figure in exam is taken from CDC which shown bats and pigs in it.
- Cycle based question is in trend. Kindly read all cycles related to viruses.

11. If blood spillage in emergency ward, what will you do first?

a. Cover with absorbent material
b. Pour hypochloride solution 1%
c. Ask the intern to mop the area
d. Wipe the surface with disinfectants

Ans. a. Cover with absorbent material.

- Spillage management protocol is (in sequential manner as mentioned below):
  - Wear gloves
    ↓
  - Cover with absorbent material
    ↓
  - Pour hypochloride 1%
    ↓
  - Leave for 30 min
    ↓
  - Clean the area
    ↓
  - Wipe surface with disinfectants
    ↓
  - Mop to leave clean area

FORENSIC MEDICINE AND TOXICOLOGY

1. Aggravated penetrative sexual assault under POCSO 2012 are all *except:*

a. Threatening
b. Gang
c. During communal or secular violence
d. By police officer

Ans. a. Threatening

(The nearest possible answer to this question. The particular terminology was not used in POCSO ACT)

Ref: The Protection of Children from Sexual offences Act, 2012 (The Gazette Of India)

- Chapter II, B of The Protection of Children from Sexual Offences Act, 2012, describes "Aggravated penetrative sexual assault and punishment" as follows:
  a. Whoever, being a police officer commits penetrative sexual assault on a child
     i. Within the limits of police station or premises.
     ii. In the premises of any station house, whether or not situated in the police station, where he is appointed.
     iii. In the course of his duties.
     iv. Where he is known or identified as a police officer.
  b. Whoever, being a member of the armed forces or security forces, commits penetrative sexual assault.
     i. Within the area where he is deployed.
     ii. In any areas under the command of the forces or armed forces
     iii. In the course of his duties or otherwise.
     iv. Where the said person is known or identified as a member of the security or armed forces.
  c. Whoever being a public servant commits such offence.
  d. Whoever being on the management or on the staff of a jail, remand home, protection home, observation home or other place of custody or care and protection established by or under any law for the first time commits such offence.
  e. Whoever being on the management or staff of a hospital, whether government or private commits such offence.
  f. Whoever being on the management or staff of an educational institution or religious institution commits such offence.
  g. Whoever commits gang penetrative sexual assault on a child.
  h. Whoever commits penetrative sexual assault on a child using deadly weapons, fire, heated substance or corrosive substance.
  i. Whoever commits penetrative sexual assault on a child causing grievous hurt or bodily harm and injury to the sexual organs of the child.
  j. Whoever commits penetrative sexual assault on a child
     i. Physically incapacitates or causes the child to become mentally ill.
     ii. In case of female child, makes her pregnant.
     iii. Inflicts the child with HIV or any other life-threatening disease or infection temporarily or permanently.

k. Whoever taking advantage of child's mental or physical disability.
l. Whoever commits penetrative sexual assault on the child more than once or repeatedly.
m. Whoever commits penetrative sexual assault on the child below twelve years old.
n. Whoever being a relative of the child through blood or adoption or marriage or guardianship or in foster care or having domestic relationship with a parent of the child living in same or shared household with the child, commits penetrative sexual assault on the child.
o. Whoever being in the ownership, management or staff of any institution providing services to the child commits penetrative sexual assault on a child.
p. Whoever being in a position of trust or authority to the child commits penetrative sexual assault on a child.
q. Whoever commits penetrative sexual assault on a child knowing the child is pregnant.
r. Whoever commits penetrative sexual assault on a child and attempts to murder the child.
s. Whoever commits penetrative sexual assault on a child in the course of communal or sectarian violence
t. Whoever commits penetrative sexual assault on a child and who has been previously convicted of and offence under this act or any sexual offence punishable under any other law.
u. Whoever commits penetrative sexual assault on a child and makes the child to strip or parade naked in public.

Whoever commits aggravated penetrative sexual assault, shall be punished with rigorous imprisonment for a term which shall not be less than ten years but which may extend to imprisonment for life and shall also be liable to fine.

2. A female found dead in her bedroom. The room was not locked from inside. Blood value of alcohol 350 mg/dL with image of face, open neck and viscera. Picture was given of bruises on neck (likely 6 penny bruises), cyanosed lip. Dissected neck with soft tissue ecchymosis. What is the cause of death?

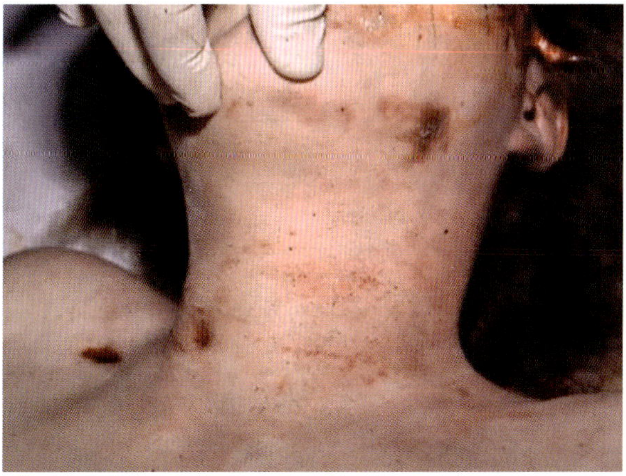

a Traumatic asphyxia
b. Café coronary
c. Throttling
d. Bansdola

Ans. c. Throttling

Traumatic asphyxia: As a result of respiratory arrest due to mechanical fixation of the chest by an unyielding substance or object, so that the normal movement of the chest wall are prevented. Due to massive compression, the chest expansion and diaphragmatic lowering are prevented. Commonly accidental in nature.

Café coronary: Seen in a healthy but grossly intoxicated person, commonly sitting in a restaurant and having a meal. He suddenly turns blue, starts coughing violently, collapses and dies. At autopsy, poorly chewed food may be seen obstructing the larynx. The high blood alcohol content anesthetises the gag reflex and causes diminished response to choked food. This is a misnomer as the cause of death is asphyxia and has got nothing to do with coronary.

Throttling: Throttling or manual strangulation is caused due to compression of neck by human hands. Death occurs due to occlusion of carotid arteries. In autopsy, small coin shaped bruises may be present caused by the assailants finger tips, which are oval to round in shape. Due to skidding of the hands of the assailants, some irregular shaped abrasions may also be present over the neck. Within the underlying neck muscles, hemorrhages or multiple petechial spots are present. Inward compression fracture of the tip of the hyoid bone may be present.

Bansdola: Type of a violent asphyxia death where a bamboo or stick is placed across the back of the neck and another across the front. Both ends are then tied by a rope and the victim is squeezed to death.

3. In the given below image, the hands present with hyperpigmentation. It occurs due to:

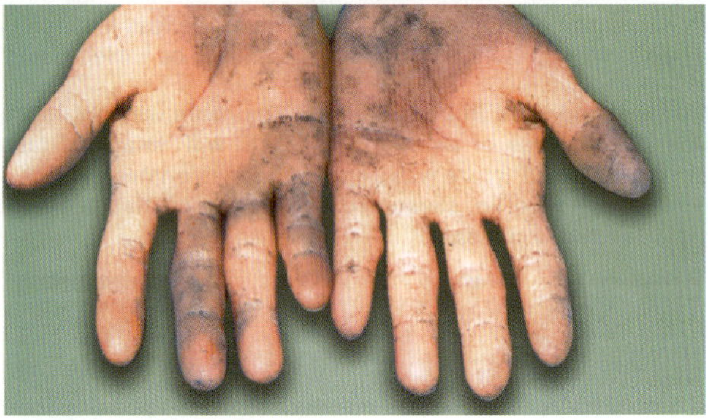

a. Chronic $CuSO_4$ poisoning
b. Long-term ingestion of arsenic water
c. Application of mercury ointment
d. Application of calotropis

Ans. b. Long term exposure of arsenic water

- *Chronic $CuSO_4$ poisoning:* chronic exposure leads to
  - *Vineyard Sprayer's lung:* Histiocytic granulomatous lung.
  - Wilson's disease.
  - Gradual anemia, green lines on gums, colic, diarrhea, peripheral neuritis, muscle atrophy.
  - Chalcosis due to deposition of copper in tissues.

- *Chronic arsenic poisoning:*
  - Polyneuritis, parestheisa, encephalopathy.
  - Rain drop pigmentation of the skin (finely mottled brown changes), involving palms, eyelids, neck.
  - Aldrich Mees line in the nails: hyperkeratosis of the palms and soles with irregular thickening of the nails and development of white transverse lines in the finger nails.
- *Chronic mercury poisoning:*
  - *Danbury tremors*: Tremors due to progressive uremia, chronic inflammation of the kidneys, GIT disturbances etc.
  - *Hatter's shake or glass blower's shake*: Seen in persons working in the hat factory. Advanced form of Danbury tremor where the tremor spreads in arms and legs.
  - *Concussio mercurialis*: No activity is possible.
  - *Mercurial erethism*: Chronic poisoning in person working at mirror manufacturing factory.
  - *Mercuriolentis*: Slit lamp examination of the eye demonstrates malt brown reflex from anterior lens capsule.
  - Renal damage with hyaline casts.
  - Acrodynia or pink disease. Idiosyncratic hypersensitivity reaction with generalized rash.
- *Calotropis*: They are organic irritants and when applied to skin causes redness and vesication.

4. In case of professional misconduct patient's records on demand should be provided within?

a. 36 hours b. 48 hours
c. 72 hours d. 7 days

Ans. c. 72 Hours

Professional misconduct is any conduct of a doctor which might reasonably be regarded as disgraceful or dishonourable. If he/she is maintaining medical record of the indoor patient for a period of three years, he/she needs to produce that record on demand in case of a professional misconduct within a period of 72 hours.

5. Within how many days a vaginal swab can be taken from a rape victim?

a. 2 days b. 3 days
c. 4 days d. 7 days

Ans. c. 4 days

Best time to detect is within 72 hours while maximum time is 96 hours

6. Concentric teeth bite mark on forearm, what to do next?

a. Two swab technique for saliva collection
b. Keep scale for measuring below the mark and take photo in the plane of bite
c. Complete description of injury as seen

Ans. a. Two swab technique for saliva collection.

7. Bullet fingerprinting is:

a. Human fingerprints on bullet b. Primary markings
c. Secondary markings d. Distorted bullet

Ans. c. Secondary markings

Bullet Fingerprinting

- Identification of the gun that fired a bullet from, an analysis of unique marks that every gun makes on the bullet it fires and on the shell ejected from it. The mechanical study of the launching, flight, behavior and effects (usually visual marks) of bullets is what ballistic fingerprinting usually refers to.
- **Synonyms are:** ballistic fingerprinting, ballistic identification
- *Secondary marking* **of bullet is called bullet fingerprint.**
- *Primary marking (Type A weapon):* Produced by manufacturing company and when bullet passed through interior of barrel of gun and 6 markings are produce due to lands called primary marking.
- Secondary marking (Type B weapon): Here only 5 lands were created due to manufacturing defect hence secondary marking for weapon of offence. So secondary marking is considered as bullet fingerprint.

8. Identify the post-mortem lividity of the image:

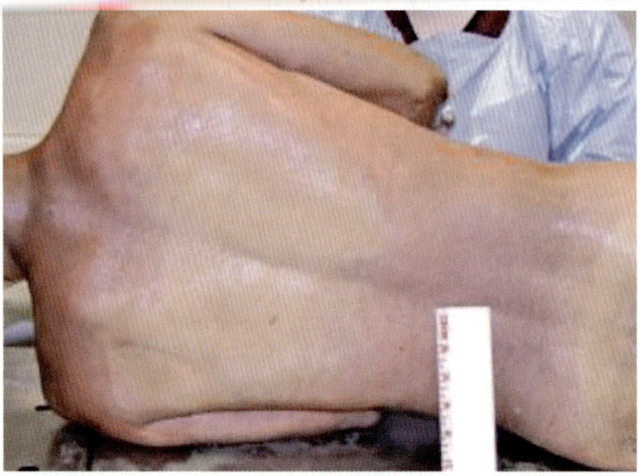

a. Tattooing b. Suggillation
c. Putrefaction d. Decomposition

Ans. b. Suggillation.

Post mortem hypostasis is the bluish-purple or purplish red discoloration which appears under the skin in the most superficial layers of the dermis (rete mucosa) due to deoxyhemoglobin, of the dependent parts of the body after death. This is due to the capillo-venous distension. Also known as post mortem staining, cadaveric lividity, suggilations, vibices and darkening of death.

Synonyms of PM Staining

- Suggillation
- PM Lividity
- PM ecchymosis
- Vibices
- Death spot
- Darkening of death
- Livor mortis

9. A 18-year-old girl was brought to OPD, labia majora separated, labia minora flabby, fourchette tear present and vagina is roomy but Hymen is intact. What could be possible?

a. Virgin
b. False virgin
c. Premenstrual stage
d. Molestation

Ans. b. False virgin

False virgin is a woman who experienced sexual intercourse.

- Hymen is intact but loose, thick and fleshy.
- Labia majora not apposing each other and not completely closing the vaginal orifice.
- Labia minora exposed and separated from majora.
- Vagina is capacious and loss of rugosity.
- Fourchette is torn and may show healed scar.
- Clitoris is enlarged.
- Posterior commissure may be torn.
- Extra genital signs like pendulous and flabby breasts, pigmented areola and nipples present.

10. Identify the lesions in the given below image:

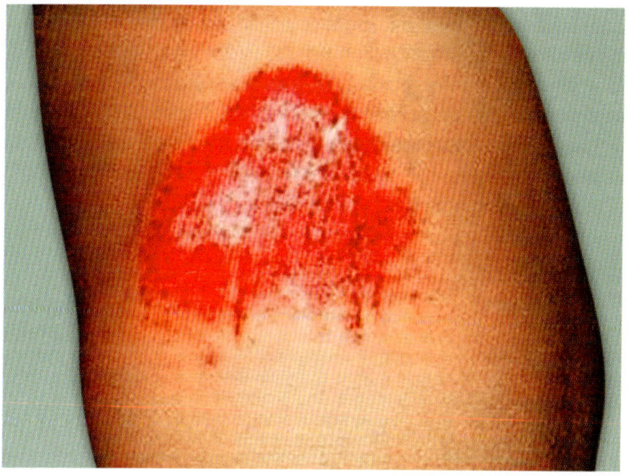

a. Abrasion
b. Laceration
c. Imprint
d. Grazes

Ans. d. Grazes

Graze abrasion is a type of abrasion, which occurs when there is movement between the skin and some rough surface in contact with it. They show uneven, longitudinal parallel lines or grooves or furrows with the epithelium heaped up at the ends of the lines, which indicate the direction in which the force was applied.

An abrasion caused by violent lateral (tangential) rubbing against a surface as in dragging over the ground is called brush burn or gravel rash.

Such phenomenon are more commonly seen in Road Traffic Accidents.

11. Identify the fracture given in the below image:

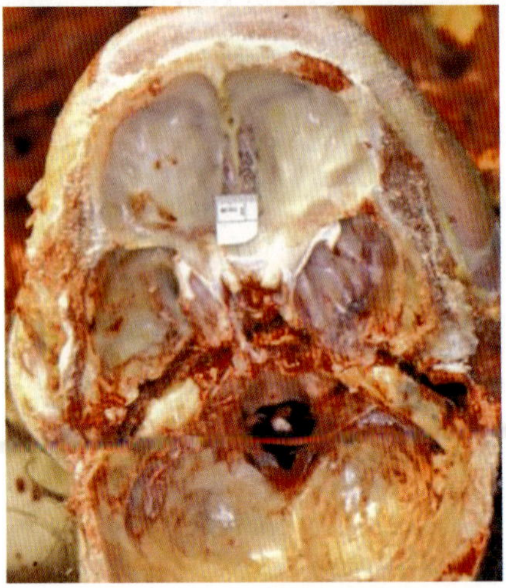

a. Pond
b. Gutter
c. Comminuted
d. Hinge fracture

Ans. d. Hinge fracture

Hinge fracture also known as motorcyclist fracture: Classical fatal injury involving both motorcyclists and pillion riders. Fracture of the skull is usually from the secondary impact with the ground. Due to a very heavy impact on one side of the head, fracture is produced across the floor of each middle fossa passing through the pituitary fossa, often associated with fissured fractures passing upwards to the temporal bones. At autopsy, the base of the skull is seen divided into two halves, each moving independently of each other like a HINGE.

ORTHOPEDICS

1. Earliest sign of compartment syndrome of leg:

a. Skin color changes
b. Loss of pulse
c. Tingling numbness
d. Pain on passive stretching of toes

Ans. d. Pain on passive stretching of toes

The earliest symptom of compartment syndrome is Worsening Pain

- It is typically out of proportion to the severity of the apparent injury and is exacerbated by passive stretching of the muscles within the compartment (e.g. for the anterior leg compartment, by passive ankle plantar flexion and toe flexion, which stretches the anterior compartment muscles).
- Compartments may feel tense when palpated.
- 6Ps:
  - Pain
  - Poikilothermia
  - Paraesthesias
  - Paralysis
  - Pallor
  - Pulselessness
- Compartment syndrome is a painful condition that occurs when pressure within the muscles builds to dangerous levels. This pressure can decrease blood flow, which prevents nourishment and oxygen from reaching nerve and muscle cells.
- Compartment syndrome can be either acute or chronic.
- Acute compartment syndrome is a medical emergency. It is usually caused by a severe injury. Without treatment, it can lead to permanent muscle damage.
- Chronic compartment syndrome, also known as exertional compartment syndrome, is usually not a medical emergency. It is most often caused by athletic exertion.

Diagnosis

- Delta pressure <= 30 mm Hg (diastolic pressure – compartment pressure)
- **Stretch test:** Earliest sign

Ref: https://orthoinfo.aaos.org/en/diseases—conditions/compartment syndrome/

2. Identify the image:

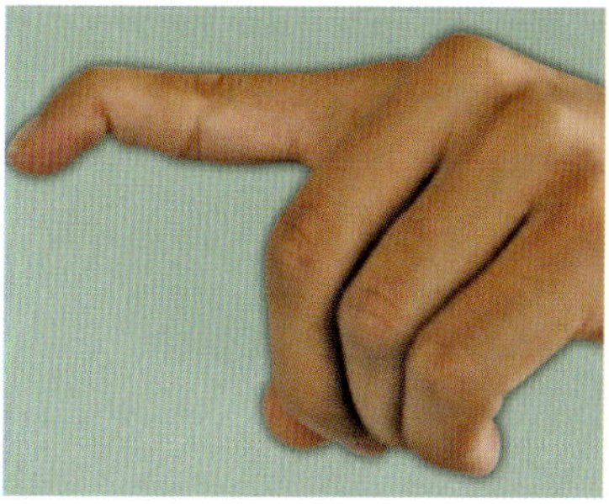

a. Mallet finger
b. Swan neck
c. Boutonniere
d. Jersey finger

Ans. a. Mallet finger

A. **Mallet finger** is a deformity of the **finger** caused when the tendon that straightens your **finger** (the extensor tendon) is damaged. When a ball or other object strikes the tip of the **finger** or thumb and forcibly bends it, the force tears the tendon that straightens the **finger**.

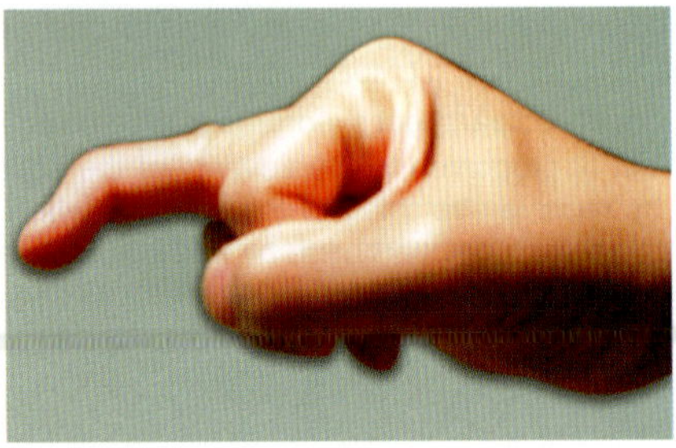

B. **Swan neck deformity** is a deformed position of the finger seen in the inflammatory condition like rheumatoid arthritis in which the joint closest to the fingertip is permanently bent toward the palm while the nearest joint to the palm is bent away from it (DIP flexion with PIP hyperextension).

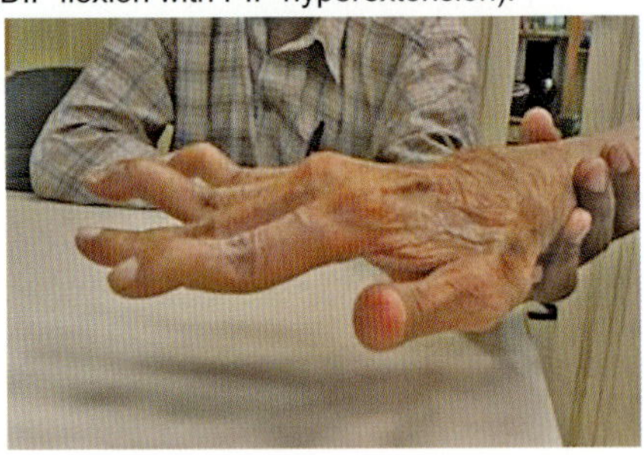

C. **Boutonniere deformity** is a deformed position of the fingers or toes also seen in the inflammatory condition like rheumatoid arthritis in which the joint nearest the knuckle (the proximal interphalangeal joint, or PIP) is permanently bent toward the palm while the farthest joint (the distal interphalangeal joint, or DIP) is bent back away (PIP flexion with DIP hyperextension).

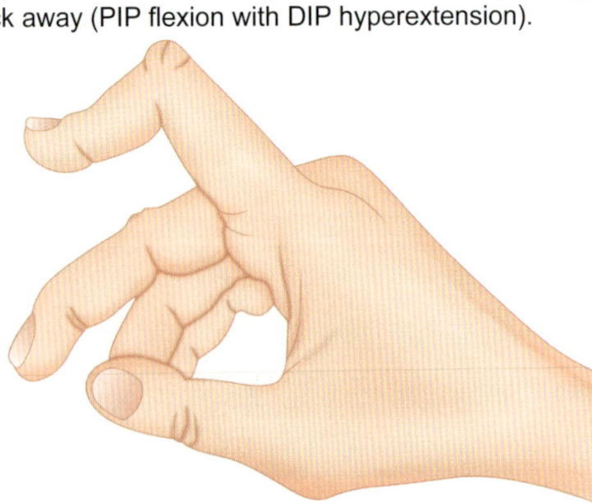

D. *Jersey finger*: A **Jersey finger** is an injury to an FDP tendon at its point of attachment to the distal phalanx. This injury often occurs in American football when a player grabs another player's jersey with the tips of one or more fingers while that player is pulling or running away.

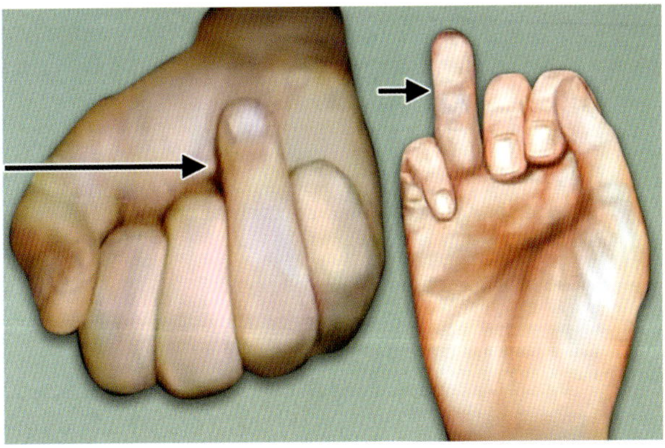

3. Patellar cluck syndrome is interposition of soft tissue at or hypertrophied scar:

a. Superior pole of patella and impinging on femoral component during flexion
b. Superior pole of patella and impinging on femoral component during extension
c. Inferior pole of patella and impinging on femoral component during flexion
d. Inferior pole of patella and impinging on femoral component during extension

Ans. b. Superior pole of patella and impinging on femoral component during extension

Definition

A painful, palpable "clunk" at the patellofemoral articulation of posterior stabilized TKA caused by a fibrous nodule of scar tissue at the posterior surface of the distal quadriceps tendon/superior patellar pole catching on the box of the femoral component during knee extension.

Epidemiology

- Prevalence reported at 3.5%
- Even less frequent with newer component designs

Component Factors

- Patellar component
- Small patellar component
- Because of decreased quads tendon contact forces against superior aspect of intercondylar box, allowing fibrosynovial proliferation and entrapment in intercondylar region of the box

- Patellar component placed low on the patella
- Exposes unresurfaced superior pole and quadriceps tendon to contact with femoral component
- Patellar over-resection and thin patellar button
- Reduces offset of quadriceps tendon from top of trochlear groove
- Exposure of cut patellar bone that is not covered by patellar component
- Resect uncovered lateral patellar facet
    - Femoral component
        - PS design
        - Increased posterior femoral condylar offset
        - Smaller femoral component
        - Femoral component in flexed position
            - Causes by more posterior entry point for intramedullary distal femoral cutting jig, because of anterior bow of femur
        - Femoral component with higher intercondylar box ratio (trochlear groove extended more proximal and anterior)
    - Thick polyethylene insert
        - Raises joint line, creates relative patella baja

Pathophysiology

- Cause of scar tissue is unknown, but may be related to:
    - Direct trauma to quadriceps tendon during patella resection during TKA
    - Impingement of the quadriceps tendon on the femoral component due to an undersized patellar component
- Scar is entrapped within the intercondylar notch during flexion
- The scar is forced out of the notch during active knee extension
- The painful snap or clunk is usually felt between 30–45 degrees
- Presents an average of 12 months after TKA
- Symptoms
    - Patellofemoral knee pain
    - Complaints of knee "popping" and "catching"
- Physical exam
    - Painful, palpable "pop" or "catch" as knee extends (~40° of flexion)
- Imaging
    - *Ultrasound:* Shows suprapatellar fibrous tissue

Treatment

Operative

- Arthroscopic vs open resection of fibrous nodule
    - Indications
    - Severe symptoms
    - Outcomes of arthroscopic resection are good, with very low rates of recurrence and improvement in knee society scores

4. An 8-year-old child presents with fever and wound with discharging pus from right thigh for 4 months. Given below is the X-ray with labelled structure. Identify:

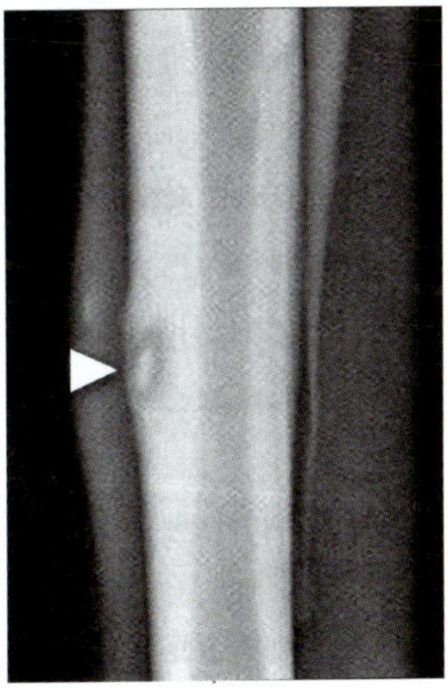

a. Sequestrum
b. Cloacae
c. Involucrum
d. Woven bone

Ans. a. Sequestrum

Chronic Osteomyelitis

- **Sequestrum** is the necrotic bone that is embedded in the pus/ infected granulation tissue.
- **Involucrum** is the new bone laid down by the periosteum that surrounds the sequestra
- **Cloaca** is the opening in the involucrum through which pus and sequestra make their way out.

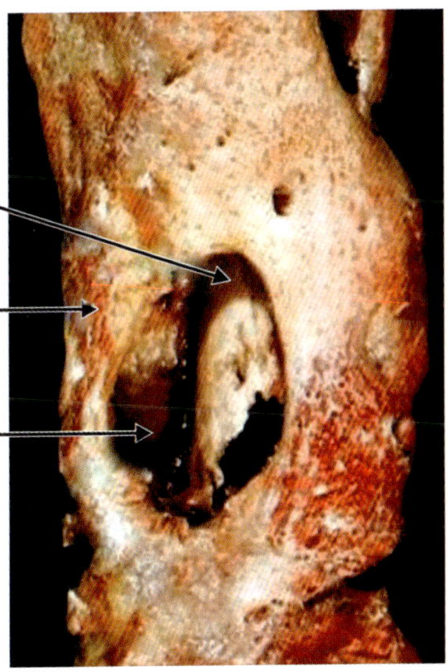

Woven bone: Haphazard organization of collagen fibers and is mechanically weak.

5. This is the X-ray of a 7-year-old child. Identify the deformity:

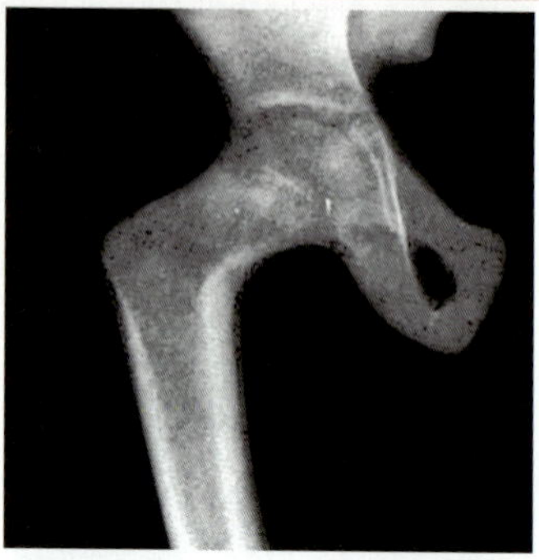

a. Coxa vara
b. Coxa valgus
c. Coxa magna
d. Coxa saltans

Ans. a. Coxa vara

Coxa Vara: Femoral neck shaft angle <120

Coxa valgus: Increased neck shaft angle >135

Coxa saltans: It is also known as snapping hip.

Snapping hip: The term "snapping hip" is used to describe any of several musculotendinous conditions associated with hip discomfort. Athletes with "snapping hip" notice an audible or palpable "snap" with certain movements. Pain may or may not accompany the sensation. The more common extra-articular causes of snapping hip involve movement of the gluteus maximus tendon, tensor fascia lata, or iliotibial band over the greater trochanter.

As symptoms are noted at the greater trochanter, this is sometimes referred to as external snapping hip. The "snapping" is produced by a combination of hip flexion, abduction, and external rotation.

In most cases of snapping hip, symptoms are minimal and there is little impact on athletic activity. In many cases, symptoms resolve with physical therapy focused on improving the function of the gluteus maximus, gluteus medius, and iliopsoas.

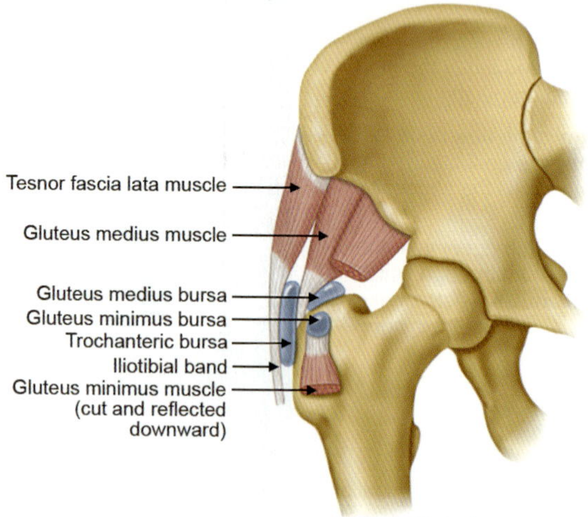

Ref : Uptodate snapping hip article

Coxa magna is the asymmetrical, circumferential enlargement and deformation of the femoral head and neck. Definitions in the literature vary but enlargement with asymmetry >10% in size is a reasonable cut-off for diagnosis.

6. Identify the well circumscribed osteolytic lesion in a 8-year-old child in the calcaneum with pigmented deposition with histopathological image:

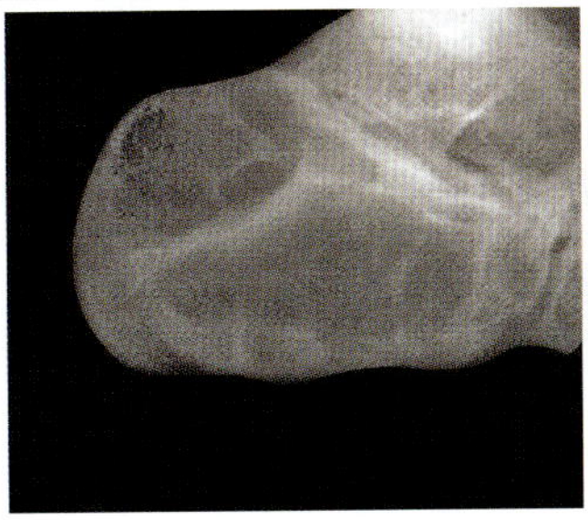

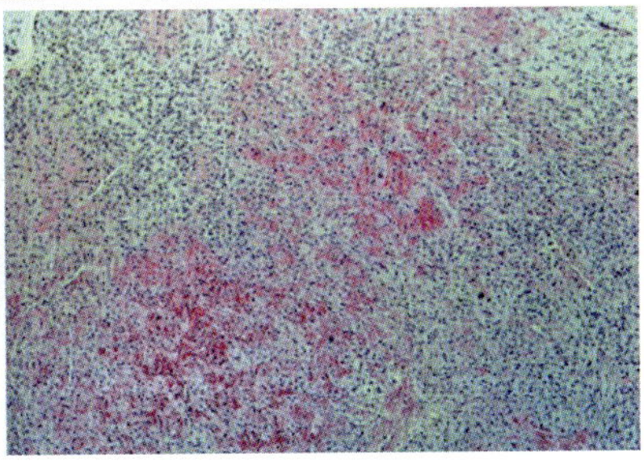

a. Ochronosis
b. Hemophilic pseudotumor
c. Pigmented villonodular synovitis
d. Eumycetes/mycetoma

Ans. b. Hemophilic pseudotumor

- Hemophilic pseudotumor is a rare complication occurring in 1–2% of patients with severe cases of hemophilia (clotting factor level, < 1% of normal)
- The pseudotumor grows as a chronic, slowly expanding, encapsulated cystic mass as a result of recurrent hemorrhage in extra-articular musculoskeletal systems. Pseudotumors are categorized as osseous and soft-tissue lesions, on the basis of anatomic location.

Diagnosis

X-ray is useful in diagnosis: Uniloculated to multiloculated lytic, expansile lesion of variable size

Ref: https://www.ajronline.org/doi/full/10.2214/ajr.183.1.1830055

7. Identify the lesion. Lytic lesion at end of radius

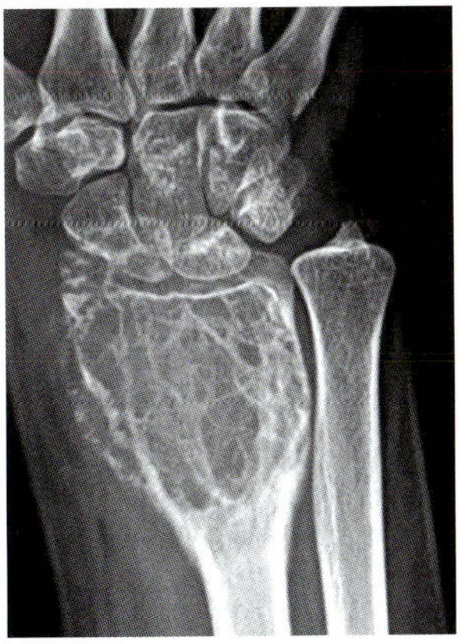

a. GCT
b. ABC (Aneurysmal bone cysts)
c. Osteoclastoma
d. Osteosarcoma

Ans. a and c. GCT and Osteoclastoma

Giant Cell Tumor

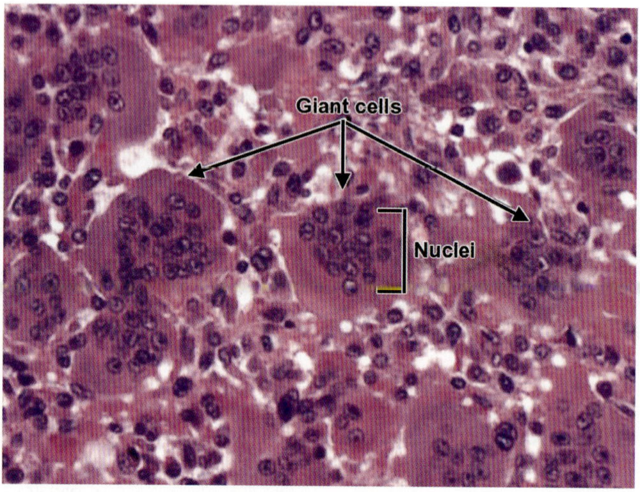

- Multinucleated giant cells that express RANKL.
- Common age group 20–40 year
- Epiphysis of long bones is most common site (often in knee region)
- M/C distal femur and proximal tibia
- Also called osteoclastoma
- Locally aggressive benign tumour. "Soap bubble" appearance on X-ray
- While in ABC lesion in metaphysis.

8. First reflex to be regained after spinal shock:

a. Abdominal reflex
b. Plantar reflex
c. Bulbocavernosus reflex
d. Cremasteric reflex

Ans. c. Bulbocavernosus reflex

If it regained after spinal shock, it shows patient is improving.

9. Which metabolic condition has phosphaturia and osteomalacia?

a. Fibrosarcoma
b. Osteosarcoma
c. Undifferentiated sarcoma
d. Malignant peripheral nerve sheath tumor

Ans. a. Fibrosarcoma

- Oncogenic (tumor-induced) osteomalacia is a rare paraneoplastic syndrome of phosphate wasting that is frequently associated with phosphaturic mesenchymal tumor (PMT)
- The differential diagnosis included a variety of benign and malignant spindle cell neoplasms: monophasic synovial sarcoma
- The bland-appearing cytologic features of a spindle cell tumor in a patient with osteomalacia should suggest the diagnosis of PMT.

Pathophysiology

Renal phosphate wasting, hypophosphatemia, decreased serum 1, 25-dihydroxy-vitamin D3 levels, and resistance to vitamin D supplementation

Clinical Feature

- Most of the patients present in their fourth decade of life
- Men and women are equally affected
- Immunohistochemical analysis has shown that PMT may be focally positive for muscle specific actin negative for CD34, S-100
- Desmin
- Chromogranin
- Neuron specific enolase
- Factor VIII-related antigen
- Leukocyte common antigen
- Cytokeratin
- Granular cytoplasmic staining with a polyclonal antibody to FGF-23

Ref: Policarpio-Nicolas, M.L., Abbott, T. E., Dalkin, A.C., Bennett-Wick, J., & Frierson, H. F. (2008). Phosphaturic mesenchymal tumor diagnosed by fine-needle aspiration and core biopsy: A case report and review of literature. Diagnostic Cytopathology, 36(2), 115–119.doi:10.1002/dc.20772

OPHTHALMOLOGY

1. A 2-year-old child watering of eyes with bilateral proptosis and photophobia, what may be the diagnosis?

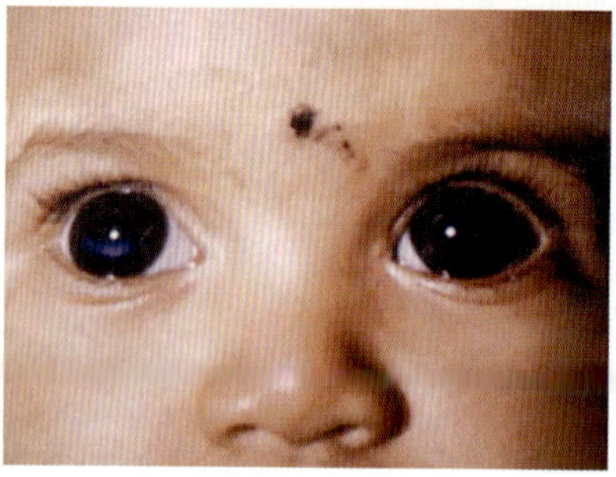

a. Congenital glaucoma
b. Retinoblastoma
c. Congenital endothelial dystrophy
d. Megalocornea

Ans. a. Congenital glaucoma

- Pointer Bilateral watering photophobia
- In Rb it will be leucocoria or strabismus and mostly unilateral
- Congenital endo dystrophy will have opaque cornea and no proptosis
- Megalocornea will not have watering and proptosis

2. Give image signifies which of the following condition?

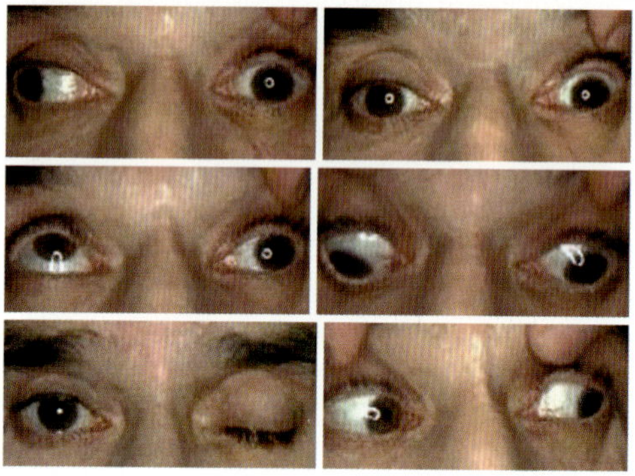

a. Internuclear ophthalmoplegia
b. Oculomotor nerve palsy
c. Lateral rectus paralysis
d. Trochlear nerve palsy

Ans. b. Oculomotor nerve palsy.

- Third nerve palsy
- Pointer-patient has ptosis in left eye with defect in all movement except abduction of left eye i.e. preserved LR

3. Most common eye manifestation in Sturge-Weber syndrome?

a. Uveitis
b. Glaucoma
c. Retinitis pigmentosa
d. Keratitis

Ans. b. Glaucoma is most common eye manifestation(one liners)

Ref: Kanski 8th edition 394

4. A patient came to AIIMS OPD, with acute pain and watering from eye for 3 days. There was 3 x 2 mm ulcer on the cornea with ROLLED OUT margins and feathery and finger like projections with minimal hypopyon:

a. Acanthamoeba
b. Pseudomonas
c. Aspergillus
d. HSV-2

Ans. d. HSV-2

- Epithelial keratitis
- Fungal can have similar description but no pain or late onset pain and vegetable matter injury history
- Acanthomoeba can have pain and watering but usually has ring like lesion
- Pseudomonas has a very fulminant course, involves and sloughed off whole cornea

Ref: Srinivasan M, Mascarenhas J, Prashanth CN. Distinguishing infective versus noninfective keratitis. Indian J Ophthalmol. 2008;56(3):203-7. this paper has the typical description

5. The spectacles in used in:

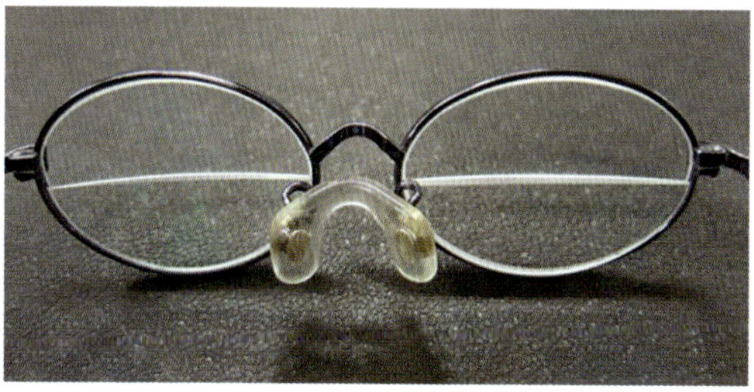

a. Progressive glasses for presbyopia
b. Bifocal glasses for presbyopia
c. Executive bifocals for pediatric pseudophakia
d. Bifocals for adult aphakia

Ans. c. Executive bifocals for pediatric pseudophakia

- The "Franklin Lens" is one of the solutions for these kinds of requests. This type of lens is a type of executive lens (Ex type lenses) in more general.
- This is a type of lens in which four pieces of lenses in total are made and combined into a single pair of lenses. All of the four lenses are single vision lenses, 2 for the far vision for both the R and L eyes, the other 2 made for the near vision of both the R and L eyes. Each of these lenses are then cut in half to be fit and fixed into a single pair of frame.
- Here below is the picture of the actual lenses. You can recognize the line in where the four lenses are combined.

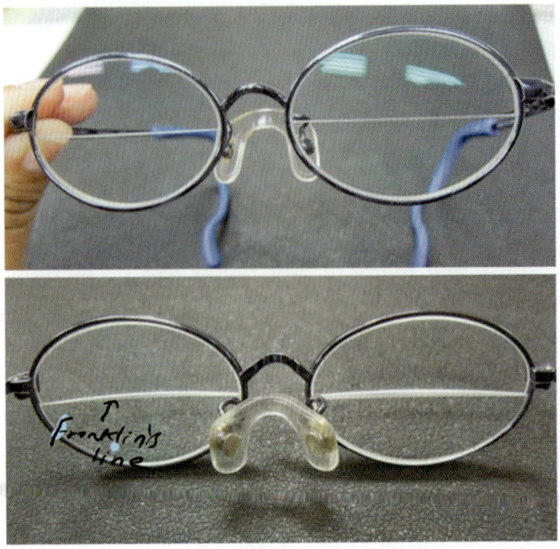

6. What is the angle subtended by the biggest letter of Snellen's chart at Nodal point of eye from 6 m:

a. 5 minutes
b. 20 minutes
c. 30 minutes
d. 60 minutes

Ans. d. 60 minutes

- Actual answer is 50 but closest one option is 60.
- Biggest letter of snellen's chart subtend 5 minute angle from distance of 60 meters, so at 6 meters it will produce 5×10 = 50.

ENT

1. A person presented to OPD with complaints of rotatory vertigo and nausea in the morning on change in position of the head. What is your diagnosis?

a. Labyrinthitis
b. BPPV
c. Vestibular neuronitis
d. Meniere's disease

Ans. b. BPPV

- BPPV is characterized by vertigo when head is placed in a certain critical position.
- There is no hearing loss.
- It is caused by disorder of posterior semicircular canal.
- Pathophysiology: Otoconial debris consisting of calcium carbonate is released from degenerating macula of utricle and floats freely in the endolymph. When it settles on cupula of posterior semicircular canal in a critical head position it causes displacement of cupula and vertigo.
- *Diagnosis:* The typical history and hallpike maneuver establishes the diagnosis.
- *Treatment:* Epley's maneuver

2. A 16-year-old male complains of nasal obstruction, nasal blockage, a mass is seen in the nasopharynx with minimal extension into sphenoid sinus. What is the stage of nasopharyngeal fibroma?

a. IA
b. IB
c. IIA
d. IIB

Ans. b. IB

- Juvenile nasoangiofibroma is a rare, benign, but locally aggressive tumor predominantly seen in adolescent males in the second decade of life.
- Diagnosis is mostly based on clinical picture.
- Investigation of choice CT scan of head with contrast enhancement.
- Surgical excision is the treatment of choice.
- For recurrent cases options are observation, revision surgery, radiation. Radiation (stereotactic gamma knife) is also used when tumor recurrence is surgically inaccessible or in intracranial extension.
- As only one sinus is involved Stage is IB.

Tumor stage	Classification
IA	Tumor limited to posterior nares and/or nasopharyngeal vault
IB	Tumor involving the posterior nares and/or nasopharyngeal vault with involvement of at least 1 paranasal sinus
IIA	Minimal lateral extension into the pterygomaxillary fossa
IIB	Full occupation of the pterygomaxillary fossa with or without superior erosion of the orbital bones
IIC	Extension into the infratemporal fossa or extension posterior to the pterygoid plates
IIIA	Erosion of the base of skull (middle cranial fossa/base of pterygoids)—minimal intracranial extension
IIIB	Extensive intracranial extension with or without extension into the cavernous sinus

Source: Adapted from Radkowski et al.

PREVENTIVE AND SOCIAL MEDICINE

1. Pick the right answer when 2 screening tests are done in series:

a. Increased sensitivity and decreased specificity
b. Increased specificity and decreased sensitivity
c. Increased sensitivity and increased specificity
d. Decreased sensitivity and decreased specificity

Ans. b. Increased specificity and decreased sensitivity

Ref: Leon Gordis, Epidemiology 5th edition page 95

	Test applied in Series	Test applied in Parallel	P
Net sensitivity	Decreases	Increases	I
Net specificity	Increases	Decreases	D
Net PPV	Increases	Decreases	
Net NPV	Decreases	Increases	

- When two sequential tests are used and those who test positive by the first test are brought in for the second test, there is a net loss in sensitivity, but a net gain in specificity, compared with either test alone. However, when two simultaneous tests are used, there is a net gain in sensitivity and a net loss in specificity, compared with either test alone.

2. The depicted image below represents:

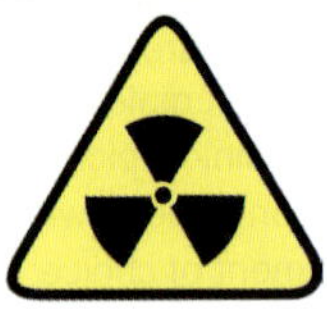

a. Biomedical waste
b. Cytotoxic waste
c. Radiation hazard
d. Bioterrorism

Ans. c. Radiation Hazard

Hazards	Symbols
Nonionizing radiation	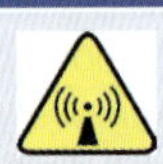
Ionizing radiation	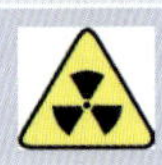
Health hazard (serious)	
Health hazard (irritant)	

Biohazard	
Toxin/poison	
Cytotoxic level	

3. In a clinical trial, blood pressure was measured between 2 independent groups following treatment, which of the following test will be suitable as at test of significance?

a. Paired t-test
b. Unpaired t-test
c. ANOVA
d. Chi-square

Ans. b. Unpaired t-test

Ref. Book of Biostatistics by V. Srinivas

Paired t-test compares study subjects at 2 different times (paired observations of the same subject). Unpaired t-test (aka Student's test) compares two different subjects. The paired t-test reduces inter-subject variability (because it makes comparisons between the same subject), and thus is theoretically more powerful than the unpaired t-test.

4. In a clinical trial, blood pressure was measured between in a group of patients before and after treatment, which of the following test will be suitable as at test significance?

a. Paired t-test
b. Mann Whitney U test
c. Student test
d. ANOVA

Ans. a. Paired t-test

Paired t-test compares study subjects at 2 different times (paired observations of the same subject). Unpaired t-test (aka Student's test) compares two different subjects. The paired t-test reduces inter-subject variability (because it makes comparisons between the same subject), and thus is theoretically more powerful than the unpaired t-test.

5. Following blood transfusion, blood bags are disposed which colour coded bin:

a. Red
b. Yellow
c. Blue
d. White

Ans. b. Yellow

Ref: http://cpcb.nic.in/cpcbold/wast/bioimedicalwast/Common_Bio_Medical_Waste_treatment_facilities.pdf

Blood bag should be discarded in yellow bin because method of disposal for yellow bag is incineration and blood bag is not made up of PVC so that blood bag can burn at safely without release of harmful gases like diaxone to environment.

Note: burning of PVC material releases diaxone (carcinogenic gas) in environment.

Method of disposal for red bin is autoclave, infected rubber and plastic waste can be thrown into red bag.

6. Which of the following true regarding the following images:

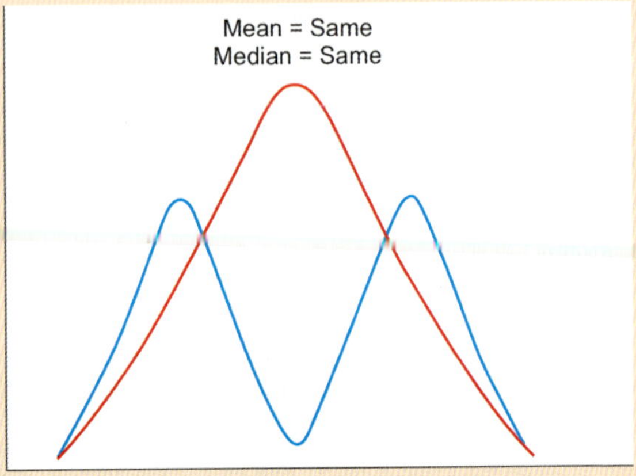

a. Mean = Median = Mode
b. Mean = Median, not equal to Mode
c. Mean = Mode, not equal to Median
d. Mean = Median and Mode are not equal

Ans. b. Mean = Median, not equal to Mode

Calculating the Mean

When you think of averaging, you are most likely to think of finding the mean. You add all of the numbers in the set and divide by how many numbers are in the list. For example, suppose you have the numbers 3, 7, 10 and 16. Add them up to get 36. Divide that number by 4 to get the average: 9.

Median: Think Middle

To determine the median, the list of numbers should be arranged in order from lowest to highest. The number in the middle, or the average of the two middle numbers, is the median. For example, if you have the numbers 1, 3, 5 and 7, the middle numbers are 3 and 5, so the median is 4.

Understanding the Mode

Mode refers to the number in a list that occurs most often. For example, in the group 12, 12, 16, 16, 16, 25 and 36, the number 16 is the mode

7. Period of isolation for measles is from:

a. Onset of catarrhal symptoms to 3 days after
b. Onset of catarrhal symptoms to 7 days after
c. Onset of catarrhal symptoms to 6 days after
d. Onset of catarrhal symptoms to 8 days after

Ans. a. Onset of catarrhal symptoms to 3 days after

Three Stages in Natural History of Measles

- *Prodormal Stage:* Begins 10 days after infection and lasts until day 14, characterized by fever, coryza, with sneezing and nasal discharge, cough, and redness of eye, lacrimation and often photophobia. A day or two before the appearance of the rash Koplik's spot like table salt crystals appear on the buccal mucosa opposite the first and second lower molars. They are small, bluish-white spots on a red base, smaller than the head of pin is pathognomonic of measles.
- *Eruptive Phase:* Characterized by dusky red, macular or maculopapular rash which begins behind the ear and spreads rapidly in few hours over the face and neck, and extends down the body taking 2-3 days to progress to lower extremities.
- Post-Measles Stage.
  - All of the following related with the following image is right; except:
  - Negatively skewed
  - Positively skewed
  - 75% values are above 25 mg
  - Median in 50 mg

Disease	Duration of isolation
Pertussis	4 weeks or until paroxysms cease
Chicken pox	Until all lesions crusted, usually about 6 days after onset of rash
Measles	From the onset of catarrhal stage through 3rd day of rash
German measles	None, except that women in the first trimester or sexually active, non-immune women in child-bearing not using contraceptive measures should not be exposed.
Cholera	3 days after tetracycline started, until 48 hours of antibiotics (or negative cultures after treatment)
Shigellosis and salmonellosis	Until 3 consecutive negative stool cultures
Polio	2 weeks adult, 6 weeks pediatric
TB (sputum+)	Until 3 weeks of effective chemotherapy
Mumps	Until swelling subsides
Meningococcal meningitis	Until the first 6 hours of effective antibiotic therapy are completed
Streptococcal pharyngitis	Until the first 6 hours of effective antibiotic therapy are completed.

8. The meal provided in mid-day meals program should supply every day:

a. One-third of energy requirement and half of the protein requirement
b. Half of energy requirement and one-third of the protein requirement
c. Half of energy requirement and half of the protein requirement
d. One third of energy requirement and one-third of the protein requirement

Ans. a. One-third of energy requirement and half of the protein requirement

- Mid-day meal scheme comes in department of education under ministry of Human Resource Development (HRD)
- Benefited up to 8th standard students
- Under mid-day meals supply: One-third of energy requirement and half of the protein requirement.

Ref.: K. Park Textbook of PSM 24th edition, page 698

9. The test used to identify frozen vaccine is:

a. Shake test b. Habel test

c. Shick test d. Test

Ans. a. Shake Test

Ref: Immunization Handbook for Medical Officers (http://nihfw.org/ pdf/ NCHRC-Publications/ImmuniHandbook.pdf)

Vaccine Damage: The physical appearance of the vaccine may remain unchanged even after it is damaged. However, the loss of potency due to either exposure to heat or cold is permanent and cannot be regained.

Freeze Damage: Hepatitis B, DPT, DT, and TT vaccines lose their potency if frozen. Freezing dissociates the antigen from the adjuvant alum thus interfering with the immunogenicity of the vaccine. Moreover, the risk of adverse events following immunization, such as sterile abscesses, may increase. Therefore, always store 'T-series' vaccines (DPT, DT, TT) and Hep.B vaccine between +2° and +8°C. If the vials are found to be frozen or contain floccules, discard the vials. Conduct the shake test, if you suspect that vials could have been frozen.

The Shake Test: The shake test is designed to determine whether adsorbed vaccines (DPT, DT, TT or Hepatitis B) have been frozen at some point of time in the cold chain. Once the vaccine is frozen it tends to form flakes which gradually settle to the bottom after the vial is shaken. Sedimentation occurs faster in a vaccine vial which has been frozen as compared to a vaccine vial which has not been frozen. Conduct the shake test if you suspect that vials could have been frozen if:

- The temperature goes below recommended ranges.
- Freeze-sensitive vaccines are stored below the basket of ILR.

Step 1: Take a vial of vaccine of the same batch number and from the same manufacturer as the vaccine you want to test, and freeze the vial until the contents are solid (at least 8 hours at -18°C). Let the vial thaw by keeping it at room temperature until it becomes liquid. Label the vial clearly so that it is easily identifiable and will not be used. Similarly label the test (suspect vial)

Step 2: Hold the “control” and “test” samples together in the same hand and shake vigorously for 10 to 15 seconds.

Step 3: Place both the vials on a table and do not move them further.

Step 4: View both vials against the light to compare their sedimentation rates.

- If the test sample shows a much slower sedimentation rate than the control sample, the test sample has most probably not been frozen and can be used.
- If the sedimentation rate is similar or more, the vial has probably been damaged by freezing and should not be used. Record the details in the stock register.

Note: Some vials have large labels which conceal the vial contents. This makes it difficult to see the sedimentation process. In such cases, turn the control and test vials upside down and observe sedimentation taking place in the neck of the vial.

Heat Damage: All vaccines are damaged by temperatures more than +8· C, whether they are exposed to a lot of heat in a short time (e.g., as a result of keeping vaccine in a closed vehicle in the sun) or a small amount of heat over a long period (e.g., as a result of the frequent opening of lid of ILR). Reconstituted BCG, measles and JE vaccines are the most sensitive to heat and light. Since these live vaccines do not contain preservatives, there is risk of contamination with staphylococcus aureus leading to Toxic Shock Syndrome and, therefore, they should not be used after 4 hours of reconstitution.

Checking for heat damage: The Vaccine Vial Monitor (VVM): A VVM is a label containing a heat-sensitive material which is placed on a vaccine vial to register cumulative heat exposure over time. The combined effects of time and temperature cause the inner square of the VVM to darken gradually and irreversibly. Before opening a vial, check the status of the VVM.
Habel Test: Use to check potency of Rabies vaccine. Schick test: Used to detect whether person susceptibility to diphtheria.

10. A health centre reports 40 to 50 cases in a week in the community. This week there are 48 cases normally. This is called?

a. Epidemic
b. Sporadic
c. Endemic
d. Outbreak

Ans. c. Endemic

Ref. Parks' Text book preventive & social medicine 24th enj; page no. 98

Endemic

- Constant presence of a disease or infectious agent in a defined geographical area.
- It is the usual or expected frequency of a disease in a population.

Epidemic

- Single exposure or point source epidemics: All cases develop within one incubation period.
- Continuous or repeated exposure epidemics: Secondary waves or peaks.
- Propagated epidemics: Results from person to person transmission.

Sporadic

- Cases which are "Scattered about"
- Cases are widely sparated in space and time
- There is no recognizable source of infection.

1. How to differentiate from Tamponade vs Tension Pneumothorax?

a. Raised JVP
b. Breath sounds
c. Raised heart rate
d. Not improving after initial fluid resuscitation

Ans. b. Breath sounds

- Best way to differentiate tamponade and tension pneumothorax in emergency is ***breath sound***.
- Breath sound absent in case of tension pneumothorax.
- Breath sound present in tamponade.
- Elevated JVP present in both situation

Pneumothorax

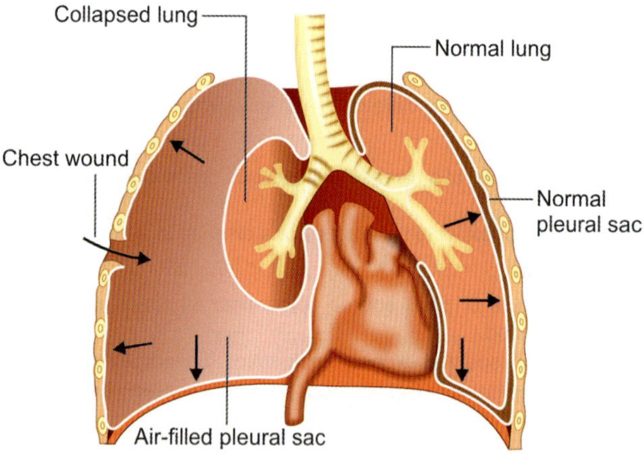

2. A patient came with a Chest trauma and Tachypnea (RR >40) and after checkup he had hypotension (BP- 90/60) and hyper-resonant note on involved side. What will be the next step?

a. Intubate
b. CXR
c. IVF
d. Wide bore needle insertion on 2nd ICS

Ans. d. Wide bore needle insertion on 2nd ICS

- **Tension pneumothorax** is classically characterized:
- Hypotension and hypoxia
- On examination: breath sounds are absent on the affected hemothorax
- Trachea deviates away from the affected side
- The thorax may also be hyper-resonant
- Jugular venous distention
- Tachycardia may be present

3. 16F Foley's color:

a. Orange
b. Blue
c. Yellow
d. Black

Ans. a. Orange

Foley's color code		
Color	**Size French**	**Size Millimeter**
Orange	6	2.0
Red	8	2.7
Yellow	10	3.3
White	12	4.0
Green	14	4.7
Orange	16	5.3
Red	18	6.0
Yellow	20	6.7
Purple	22	7.3
Blue	24	8.0
Black	26	8.7

4. Reason for thyroid storm after thyroid surgery:

a. Infection
b. Inadequate preoperative preparation
c. Thyroiditis
d. Rough handling of thyroid at surgery

Ans. b. Inadequate preoperative preparation

- Inadequate preoperative preparation is commonest cause.
- Thyroid storm is a rare, life-threatening condition characterized by severe clinical manifestations of thyrotoxicosis
- Although thyroid storm can develop in patients with longstanding untreated hyperthyroidism
- It is often precipitated by an acute event such as thyroid or nonthyroidal surgery, trauma, infection, an acute iodine load, or parturition.
- *Symptoms and signs:* Cardiovascular symptoms in many patients include tachycardia to rates that can exceed 140 beats/minute and congestive heart failure.

Hypotension

Cardiac Arrhythmia

- *Hyperpyrexia:* 104 to 106°F
- Agitation, anxiety, delirium, psychosis, stupor, or coma are also common
- Laboratory findings—All patients with overt primary hyperthyroidism have low TSH and high free T4 and/or T3 concentrations
- Other nonspecific laboratory findings may include mild hyperglycaemia, mild hypercalcemia, abnormal liver function tests, leucocytosis, or leukopenia
- Hyperglycemia is secondary to a catecholamine-induced inhibition of insulin release and increased glycogenolysis.
- Hypercalcemia may occur due to haemoconcentration and enhanced bone resorption.

Initial Approach

A beta blocker to control the symptoms and signs induced by increased adrenergic tone

- A thionamide to block new hormone synthesis
- An iodine solution to block the release of thyroid hormone
- An iodinated radiocontrast agent (if available) to inhibit the peripheral conversion of T4 to T3
- Glucocorticoids to reduce T4-to-T3 conversion, promote vasomotor stability, and possibly treat an associated relative adrenal insufficiency
- Bile acid sequestrants may also be of benefit in severe cases to decrease enterohepatic recycling of thyroid hormones

5. Nobel prize for medicine/physiology in 2018 for the discovery of:

a. Apoptotic pathway b. CRISPR-Cas9
c. Negative immune regulation
d. Molecular mechanisms controlling circadian rhythm

Ans. c. Negative immune regulation

Ref. Novel prize jointly to ***James P. Allison and Tasuku Honjo***

For their discovery of cancer therapy by inhibition of negative immune regulation. The **CRISPR/Cas 9** system was first exploited by Danisco in 2008. Technique that allows for the highly specific and rapid modification of DNA in a genome, the complete set of genetic instructions in an organism.

6. Cannot be diagnosed without positive ANA:

a. SLE b. Sjögren
c. Drug induced lupus d. Scleroderma

Ans. c. Drug induced lupus

- Drug induced lupus has 100% sensitivity for ANA
- Sensitivity of ANA for various disease:
  - SLE >95%
  - Drug induced lupus 100%
  - Sjögren 40-70%
  - Discoid lupus 15%
- Non rheumatic condition:
  - Primary autoimmune cholangitis 100%
  - Autoimmune hepatitis 100%

7. Infertility in karatgener:

a. Oligospermia b. Blockage of epididymis
c. Asthenozoospermia d. Undescended testes

Ans. c. Asthenozoospermia

- Kartagener syndrome: (Primary ciliary dyskinesia, AR)
- Bronchiectasis
- Situs-inversus
- Sinusitis
- Lack of ciliary activity interferes with bacterial clearance which predisposes the sinus and bronchi to infection.
- Affects cell motility during embryogenesis resulting in situs inversus.
- In males Most men with PCD have living but immotile spermatozoa and are infertile.

Ref: Robbins and Cotran, pathologic basis of disease page 692

8. While measuring blood pressure of a cardiac tamponade patient, what advice will you give him:

a. Hold breath
b. Breathe normally
c. Long and deep breathing
d. Short and shallow breaths

Ans. b. Breathe normally

Pulses paradoxus measurement

- To measure pulsus paradoxus, a manually-operated sphygmomanometer is employed for blood pressure measurement in the standard fashion except that the cuff is deflated more slowly than usual.
- During deflation, the first Korotkoff sounds are audible with heart beats occurring only during expiration.
  - With further cuff deflation, Korotkoff sounds become audible on all heart beats throughout the respiratory cycle.
- The difference between the systolic pressure at which the first Korotkoff sounds are heard during expiration and the pressure at which they are heard throughout the respiratory cycle quantifies pulsus paradoxus.
- Severe pulsus paradoxus, variably defined as >10 to 20 mmHg, can be palpated in the radial, brachial, or femoral pulses as a weakening or disappearance of the pulse during inspiration
- Since the depth of respiration influences the severity of pulsus, the patient should not be instructed to change his/her breathing pattern during this evaluation.

9. A 60-year-old female patient has left sided weakness since 1 hr and left sided facial weakness with BP, 160/100 mm Hg. The CT scan is normal, what is the best next step?

a. Start thrombolysis
b. Give loading dose of aspirin and clopidogrel
c. Manage BP alone
d. No interventions needed

Ans. a. Start thrombolysis

- The First step is NCCT head to rule out haemorrhagic stroke.
- As above CT head is normal, suggestive of non-haemorrhagic stroke.
- Window period for thrombolysis is <4.5 hour so this patient can be considered for thrombolysis with Alteplase/Tenecteplase.
- Thrombolytic agent, recombinant t-PA can be use between 3-4.5 hours after the onset of stroke.

Absolute contraindications	Relative contraindications
Major trauma, surgery, head trauma within 3 weeks	Cancer Age > 75-80
Prior hemorrhagic stroke	Transient ischemic attack within 6 months
Ischemic stroke within prior 6 months	Oral anticoagulant therapy
Central nervous system neoplasm	Noncompressible punctures
Gastrointestinal bleeding within one month	Traumatic resuscitation
Active bleeding	Refractory hypertension
	Advanced liver disease
	Infective endocarditis
	Active peptic ulcer
	Pregnancy or within one week postpartum

10. ECG with "mean" axis of 90°. In which lead there would be the maximum voltage of R wave?

a. III
b. I
c. aVF
d. aVL

Ans. c. aVF

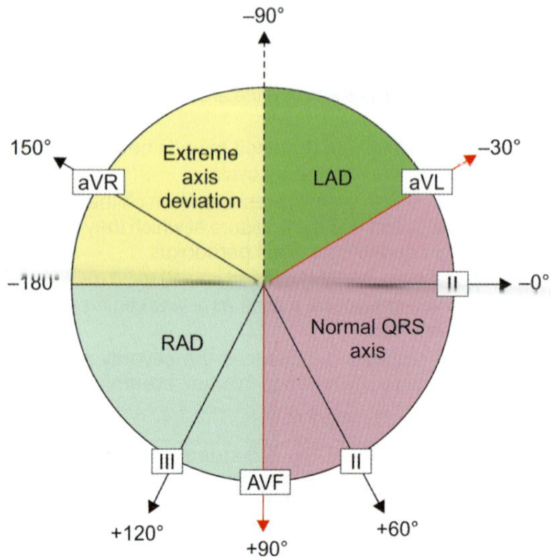

The cardiac axis of +90° corresponds to aVF thus maximum R-wave amplitude would seen in aVF only.

11. Which of the following is not done before ABG:

a. Allen's test
b. Heparin to rinse the syringe
c. Flexion of wrist
d. Poking at 45° angle

Ans. c. Flexion of wrist

- *Arterial sampling*: Arterial blood is required for an ABG.
- *Needle puncture*: Percutaneous needle puncture via needle stick or via arterial catheterization with a indwelling catheter.
- *Site selection*: Common sites include the radial ***(most common)***, femoral, dorsalis pedis, or axillary artery.
  - *Radial artery*: The radial artery is best palpated between the distal radius and the tendon of the flexor carpi radialis when the wrist is extended.
  - *Dorsalis pedis*: The dorsalis pedis artery can be occluded by the forefinger followed by compression of the nail bed of the great toe and the needle can be inserted at a ***30 degree angle*** lateral to the extensor tendon at the level of the midfoot.
- ***Ensure collateral circulation:*** Major risk associated with arterial puncture is ischemia distal to the puncture site. Thus identifying collateral flow to the region supplied by the artery can be used by clinicians prior to puncture.
  - *Modified Allen's test:* The patient's hand is initially held high with the fist clenched. Both the radial and ulnar arteries are compressed firmly by the two thumbs of the investigator.

Modified Allen's Test

- The radial and ulnar arteries are occluded by firm pressure while the fist is clenched until the hand blanches

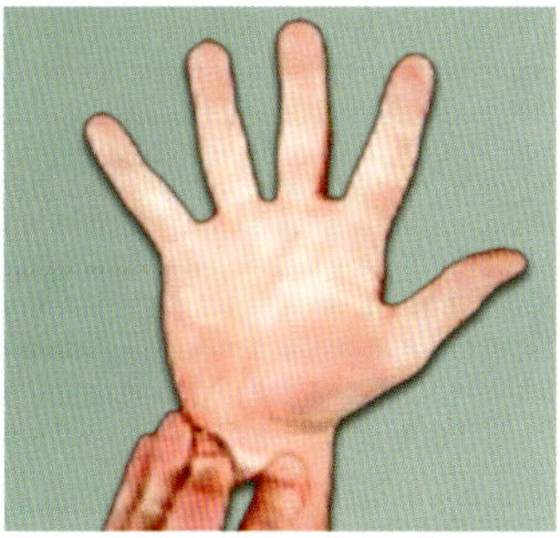

- The hand is opened and the pressure is released from the ulnar artery

- Colour should return within 15 seconds to imply adequate arterial circulation

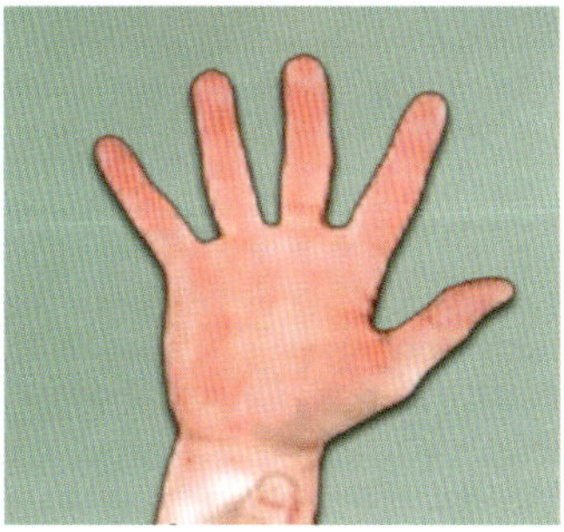

- *The Allen's test*: The Allen's test (from which the modified Allen's test evolved).

Technique

Once a palpable artery has been located, blood is withdrawn using the following steps.

- The planned puncture site should be sterilely prepared.
- Local analgesia with injectable 1 to 2 percent lidocaine can be administered but is not usually performed.
- On extended wrist then gently palpate the artery in one or two fingers while holding the needle in the other hand.
- Radial artery and dorsalis pedis should be punctured with the needle at a 30 to 45 degree angle.
- Femoral artery should be punctured at a 90 degrees angle (femoral artery).

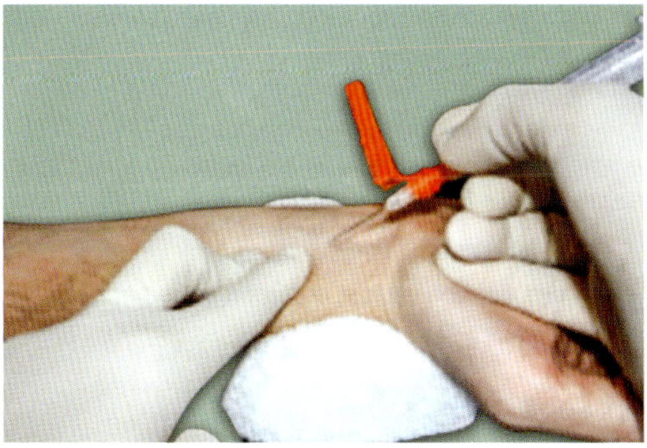

- Heparinization of syringe

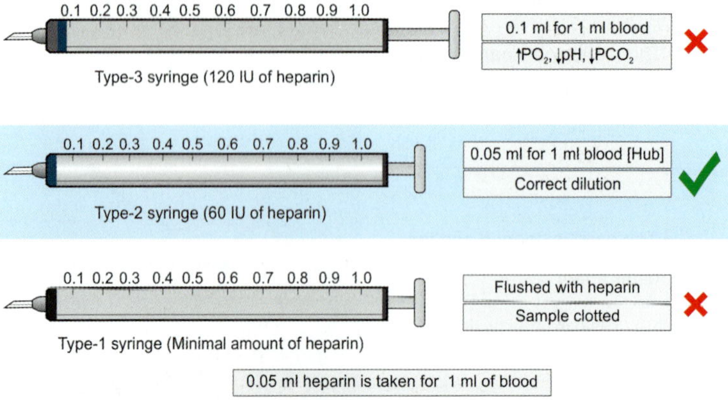

***ABG interpretation is very important for AIIMS** [illegible]

12. Patient had recurrent optic neuritis of both eyes with extensive transverse myelitis. Visual acuity in right eye is 6/60 and visual acuity in left eye 6/18. Patient showed 50% response to steroids. Diagnosis is:

a. Neuromyelitis optica (NMO)
b. Subacute combined degeneration of spinal cord (SACD)
c. Posterior cerebral artery stroke
d. Neurosyphilis

Ans. a. Neuromyelitis optica (NMO)

- Acute transverse myelitis (ATM) is a rare acquired neuro-immune spinal cord disorder.
- This has a rapid onset of weakness, sensory alterations, and bowel or bladder dysfunction.

Classification

- Acute partial TM refers to spinal cord dysfunction that is mild or grossly asymmetric with an MRI lesion extending one to two vertebral segments.
- Acute complete TM refers to spinal cord dysfunction that causes symmetric, complete or near complete neurologic deficits (paresis, sensory loss, and autonomic dysfunction) below the level of the lesion with an MRI lesion extending one to two vertebral segments.
- Longitudinally extensive transverse myelitis (LETM) refers to complete or incomplete spinal cord dysfunction with a lesion on MRI that extends three or more vertebral segments.

Aetiology

- Postinfectious complication—Most common cause of ATM;
  - HIV myelopathy
  - HSV 2
  - Varicella zoster
  - Ebstein-barr virus

- Neuro-inflammatory disorders—
  - Acute disseminated encephalomyelitis(ADEM),
  - Multiple sclerosis, and
  - Neuromyelitis optica(NMO).
  - Autoimmune – SLE, Sarcoidosis, Sjogren's syndrome, Behcet's Disease
  - Vascular – AV malformations
  - Neoplastic –paraneoplastic syndromes
  - Metabolic --SACD

Treatment

Intravenous glucocorticoids have long been considered the standard of care and first-line therapy in acute idiopathic TM.

Neuromyelitis Optica (NMO)

- Combination of optic neuritis and ATM.
- Spinal cord lesion length important distinguishing factor between NMO and MS
- Longitudinally extensive transverse myelitis (LETM) refers to idiopathic spinal cord inflammatory lesions extending more than three vertebral segments on the MRI.
- NMO-IgG seropositivity appears to be much more likely in patients with LETM.
- Longitudinally extensive transverse myelitis was seen in 51% and included all cases of NMO, ATM, and recurrent ATM.

Neurosyphilis Associated Myelopathy

- Most common manifestation ATM, followed by chronic myelopathy
- Presents with features of chronic myelopathy –in the form of dorsal myelopathy and one presented with features like motor neuron disease.

Neurosarcoidosis

- The most common presenting symptoms were lower extremity weakness and paresthesias.
- Thoracic segment was most frequently involved (80%). Lesions were mostly intramedullary and nearly half involved the leptomeninges.
- Angiotensin-converting enzyme levels in cerebrospinal fluid were elevated but not confirmatory.

Subacute Combined Degeneration (SACD)

- Vitamin B12 deficiency leads to degeneration of the dorsal and lateral white matter of the spinal cord, producing a slowly progressive weakness, sensory ataxia, and paresthesias, and ultimately spasticity, paraplegia, and incontinence
- Supplemental treatment with vitamin B12 Stop progression and improve neurologic deficits in most patients

13. A patient who is a known case of CKD has complaints of vomiting. His ABG reports are as follows: pH – 7.40, pCO_2 – 40, HCO_3 – 25, Na – 145, chloride-100.

a. Normal anion gap met acidosis
b. High anion gap met acidosis
c. No acid base abnormality
d. High anion gap metabolic acidosis with metabolic alkalosis

Ans. d. High anion gap metabolic acidosis with metabolic alkalosis

Basic steps in Analysis of ABG

Validate ABG

- The $[H^+]$ obtained from the pH of the ABG should be equal to that calculated from **Kassirer- Bleich equation: $(H^+) = 24 \times PCO_2/(HCO_3^-)$** the ABG to be valid.
- Calculated $H^+ = 24(CO_2)/HCO_3^-$
- Actual $H^+ = (7.80 - pH) \times 100$

Question

- Calculated $H^+ = 24(40)/25$ = approx—40
- Actual $H^+ = (7.80 - 7.40)(100) = 40$

Assess Oxygenation

Alveolar-arterial Oxygen Gradient (A-a gradient):

Alveolar gas equation

- A – a gradient = $PAO_2 - PaO_2$
- $PAO_2 = FIO_2 (P_{atm} - P_{H_2O})) - PaCO_2 \times 1/RQ$
  $= 0.21(760–47) - PCO_2/0.8$

On room air (0.21× (760–47) = 149.7 mm Hg thus,

A— a gradient is approximated as: $[150 - 5/4(pCO_2)] - Pa_{o2}$ at sea level

- Normal 5 to 10 mm Hg
- Needs age and FiO_2 correction
- Age/4+4
- ↑5-7 mm Hg every 10% ↑in FiO_2

- Helps to differentiate between the two mechanisms of hypoxemia.
- If the A-a gradient is normal—either hypoventilation and low atmospheric.
- If the A-a gradient is decreased then either shunt physiology or V/Q mismatch.

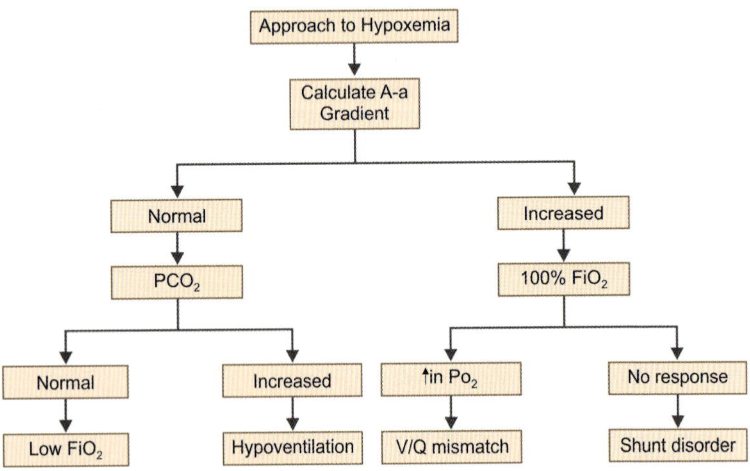

V/Q vs shunt disorder

Shunt	
❑ ARDS ❑ Pneumonia ❑ Pulmonary edema ❑ Pulmonary AVM	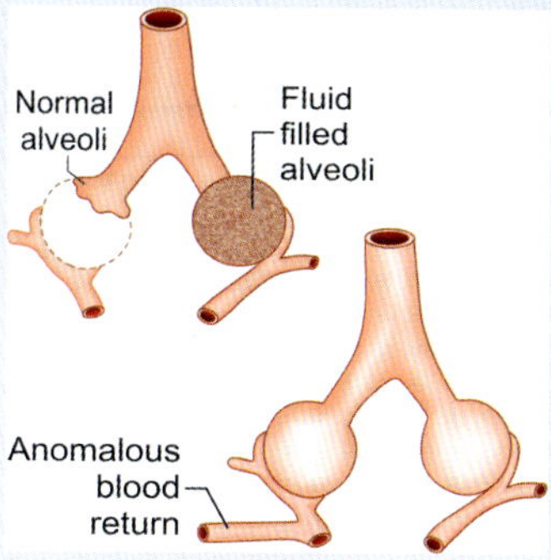
V/Q Mismatch	
❑ Emphysema ❑ ILD ❑ Pulmonary vascular disease ❑ Positive pressure ventilation	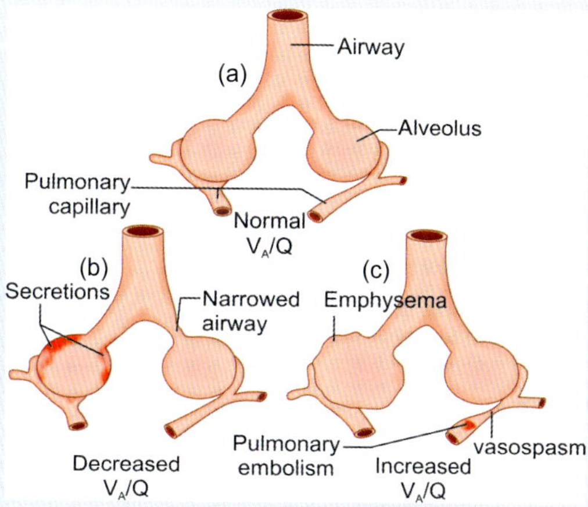

Not required here.

pH: Acidemic or Alkalemic?

Acid base status is defined in terms of the plasma pH.

Acidemia: Decrease in the blood pH below normal range of 7.35–7.45.

Alkalemia: Elevation in blood pH above the normal range of 7.35–7.45.

Acidosis: Process that increases [H+] by increasing PCO_2 or by reducing $[HCO_3^-]$

Alkalosis: Process that reduces [H+] by reducing PCO_2 or by increasing $[HCO_3^-]$

Primary disorder: Metabolic or Respiratory?

Characteristics of 1° Acid-base disorder

Kassirer-Bleich equation : $H^+ = \dfrac{24 \times (PCO_2)}{(HCO)_3^-}$

Disorder	Primary responses			Compensatory response
Metabolic acidosis	↑ (H^+)	↓ pH	↓ HCO_3^-	PCO_2
Metabolic alkalosis	↓ (H^+)	↑ pH	↑ HCO_3^-	↑ PCO_2
Respiratory acidosis	↑ (H^+)	↓ pH	↑ pCO_2	↑ HCO
Respiratory alkalosis	↓ (H^+)	↑ pH	↓ pCO_2	↓ HCO_3^-

If respiratory disorder: Acute or Chronic?

Expected Compensation

For Metabolic Acidosis: Calculate Anion Gap

Anion gap: 145-(100+24)= 21—High AG

For high-AG metabolic acidosis →calculate Delta gap?

- *Delta gap* = (HCO_3^-) + (AG – 12)
  - If < 24, patient has an additional non-anion gap metabolic acidosis
  - If >24, patient has an additional **metabolic alkalosis** (In question).
- *Delta gap*: 24+(21-12)= 33
- Even with normal pH patient can have mixed acid base disorder.

14. What is the best marker in KDIGO criteria to differentiate renal from prerenal AKI?

a. Urinary Na
b. Urinary NGAL
c. $U_{Na} \times S_{cr} / S_{Na} \times U_{cr}$
d. a U_{osm}

Ans. c. $U_{Na} \times S_{cr} / S_{Na} \times U_{cr}$

Acute Kidney Injury (AKI)

- Abrupt Loss of Kidney Function, resulting in the retention of urea and other nitrogenous waste products and in the dysregulation of extracellular volume and electrolytes.
- The term AKI has largely replaced acute renal failure (ARF),
  - In 2004, the Acute Dialysis Quality Initiative (ADQI) group proposed a consensus graded definition, called the RIFLE criteria
  - A modification of the RIFLE criteria was subsequently proposed by the Acute Kidney Injury Network (AKIN, which included the ADQI group)
  - More recently, the Kidney Disease: Improving Global Outcomes (KDIGO)

Kdigo Modifications to Rifle and Akin

The kidney disease: Improving Global Outcomes (KDIGO) Clinical Practice Guidelines for AKI included a revision to the definition of AKI while retaining the Acute Kidney Injury Network (AKIN) staging criteria.

In the Kdigo Definition

- The timeframe for an absolute increase in serum creatinine of ≥0.3 mg/dL is retained from the AKIN definition (48 hours)
- While the timeframe for a ≥50 percent increase in serum creatinine reverted to the seven days originally included in the Acute Dialysis Quality Initiative (ADQI) RIFLE criteria.

According to KDIGO, AKI is defined by any of the following:

- Increase in serum creatinine by ≥0.3 mg/dL (≥26.5 micromol/L) within 48 hours; or
- Increase in serum creatinine by ≥1.5 times baseline, which is known or presumed to have occurred within the prior seven days; or
- Urine volume <0.5 mL/kg/h for six hours

The KDIGO criteria only utilize

- Changes in serum creatinine and urine output
- Not changes in glomerular filtration rate (GFR) for staging
- With the exception of children under the age of 18 years, for whom an acute decrease in estimated GFR (eGFR) to <35 mL/min per 1.73 m^2 is included in the criteria for stage 3 AKI.

Renal Failure Indices

Diagnostic index	Prerenal AKI	ATN
Plasma BU/Creatinine	>20	<10-15
Renal failure index (= UNa/Ucr/Pcr)	<1	<1
FE_{Na} (= Una × Pcr/Pna × Ucr)—most sensitive	<1	>1
Urine [Na+] (mEq/l)	<20	> 40
Urine urea nitrogen/Plasma urea nitrogen	>8	<3
Urine creatinine/Plasma creatinine	>40	<20
Urine Osmolality	> 500	300
Urine sediment	Hyaline casts	Muddy brown granular casts

- Several indices have been used to help differentiate prerenal azotemia from intrinsic AKI when the tubules are malfunctioning.

Utility of FE_{Na} & U_{Na} in AKI

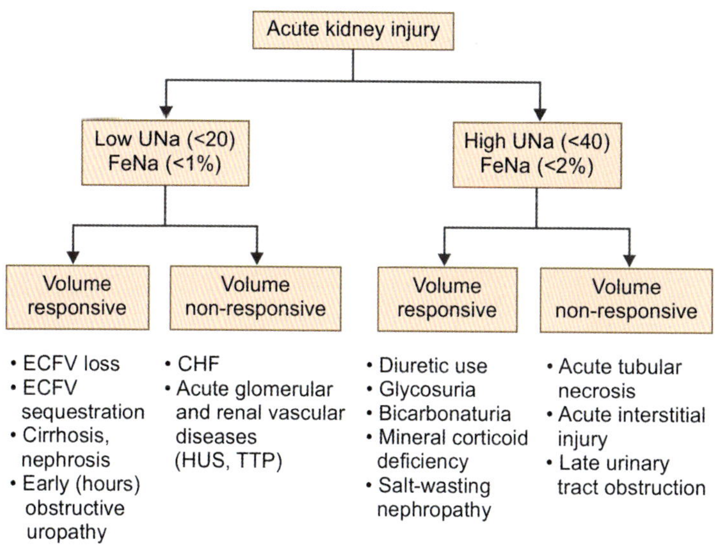

Novel Biomarkers

New Biomarkers for Detecting AKI Post Injury in Various Clinical Situations					
Bio-marker	**Sample Source**	**Cardiopulmonary Bypass (CPS)**	**Contrast Nephropathy**	**Sepsis or ICU**	**Kidney Transplant (tx)**
Cystatin C	Plasma	12 hrs post-CPS	8 hrs post-contrast	48 hrs before AKI	Variable
IL-18	Urine	4-6 hrs post-CPS	Not tested	48 hrs before AKI	12-24 hrs post-tx
KIM-1	Urine	12-24 hrs post- CPS	Not tested	Not tested	Not tested
NGAL	Urine/ Plasma	2 hrs post-CPS	2-4 hrs postcontrast	48 hrs before AKI	12-24 hrs post-tx urine only)

New Biomarkers for AKI in Various Clinical Situations

In addition to serum creatinine, there are several emerging biomarkers that offer promise for AKI. Of the potential biomarkers for AKI in various clinical situations, NGAL is one of the earliest biomarkers for AKI in various clinical settings. In the table shown in the slide, "48 hrs before AKI" indicates that the marker is elevated 48 hours before a significant rise in serum creatinine, which was used as the standard for AKI.

Abbreviations:

IL-18, interleukin-18; KIM-1, kidney injury molecule 1.

**Novel biomarker not approved by any guidelines.

Epidemiology of AKI

AKI complicates

- Acute care hospital admissions—5–7%
- Intensive care unit admissions—30%,
- Hospital mortality rates may exceed 50%.

AKI maybe community acquired or hospital-acquired.

Most Common causes of community-acquired AKI include:

- Volume depletion
- Adverse effects of medications, and
- Obstruction of the urinary tract.

The most common cause for hospital-acquired AKI include:

- Sepsis and shock(MCC),
- Major surgical procedures,
- Critical illness involving heart or liver failure,
- Contrast induced,
- Nephrotoxic medication administration.

AKI etiologies may be are region-specific such as

- **Envenomations** from snakes, spiders, caterpillars, and bees;
- **Tropical infections** the most common causes: Scrub typhus, malaria, salmonellosis, dengue and leptospirosis
- **Crush injuries** and resultant rhabdomyolysis from earthquakes.

15. Death due to smoke inhalation is due to:

a. Hypoxemia b. Anemic hypoxia
c. Ischemic hypoxia d. All of the above

Ans. d > b > a. All of the above > Anemic hypoxia > Hypoxemia

Let's First see Types of Hypoxia

- *Hypoxic hypoxia*: Limited oxygen in the environment. Divers, aviators, mountain climbers, and fire fighters are all at risk for this kind. Choking, strangulation, the crushing of the windpipe all cause this sort of hypoxia. Severe asthmatics may also experience symptoms of hypoxic hypoxia.
- *Anemic or Hypemic hypoxia*: Inadequate oxygen in the blood despite adequate environmental oxygen. Anemia and carbon monoxide poisoning are common causes of hypemic hypoxia.
- *Ischemic hypoxia (or "stagnant hypoxia"):* Inadequate blood flow to the tissue. Like shock and cardiac arrest may cause stagnant hypoxia.
- *Histotoxic hypoxia:* Oxygen is present in but the tissue but cannot be metabolized by the brain tissue. Cyanide poisoning is a well-known example.

Smoking Inhalation Injury

Pathophysiology

There are three mechanisms of smoke-induced injury (these may co-exist within one patient or occur in isolation)

- Heat
- Particulate matter deposition and respiratory irritants
- Asphyxiation and systemic toxicity

Heat

Proximal burns of the nasal and oropharyngeal mucosa are common. The smoke containing superheated steam can cause pulmonary damage, but usually this insult also causes glottic swelling/erythema and is rapidly fatal (first 24–36 h post-injury).

Particulate matter and respiratory irritants

- The main cause of pulmonary damage is by inhalation of particulate matter, mainly carbonaceous particles containing toxic chemicals (soot).
- The formation of nitric oxide, a potent vasodilator, from induced nitric oxide synthase in respiratory tissues, leads to increased bronchial blood flow, decreased hypoxic pulmonary vasoconstriction in poorly ventilated areas of lung, and results in **V/Q mismatch and hypoxia (stagnant hypoxia)**.

Systemic Toxicity

- This leads to tissue hypoxia can be caused by many mechanisms.
- Combustion utilizes oxygen thus decrease inspired oxygen concentrations as low as 10–13%—low PaO_2—hypoxic hypoxia.
- Products of incomplete combustion lead to formation of main toxic compound in fire deaths is carbon monoxide (CO) and Hydrogen cyanide.
- Hydrogen cyanide is a colourless gas with a bitter almond odour which only 40% of the population are able to detect.
- ***Carbon monoxide is one of the most frequent immediate causes of death following inhalation injury—Anemic hypoxia .***
- The presence of CO and cyanide has a synergistic effect of asphyxia.

16. Patient presents with recent onset breathlessness and ECG is taken. ECG is shown below. What is the diagnosis?

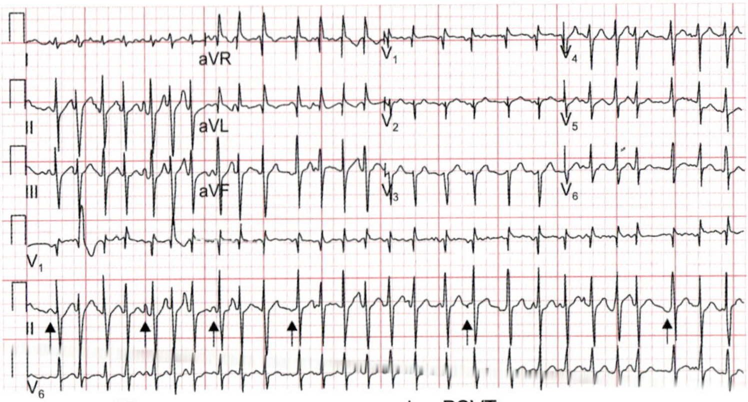

a. AF
b. PSVT
c. AMI
d. MAT

Anw. d. MAT

- **Firstly important to assess the QRS duration to classify arrhythmias in NCT and WCT.**
- **QRS duration <120 msec** — NCT i.e. ventricle are being activated via the normal His-Purkinje system i.e. origin usually SVT
- **QRS duration> 120 msec**— WCT – s/o – VT – (with some exceptional types of SVT)

Systematic Approach

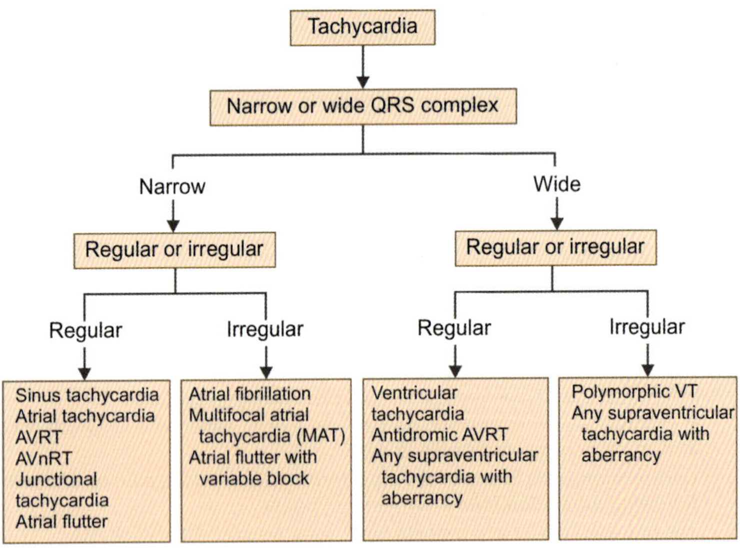

- VT often carries a much graver prognosis and therefore requires immediate attention and measures to revert to sinus rhythm.
- SVT is not usually lethal and often does not result in hemodynamic collapse; therefore, more conservative measures can be applied initially to convert to sinus rhythm.
- Therefore WCT is used when precise arrhythmia mechanism cannot be determined.

Approach to Narrow Complex Tachycardia (NCT)

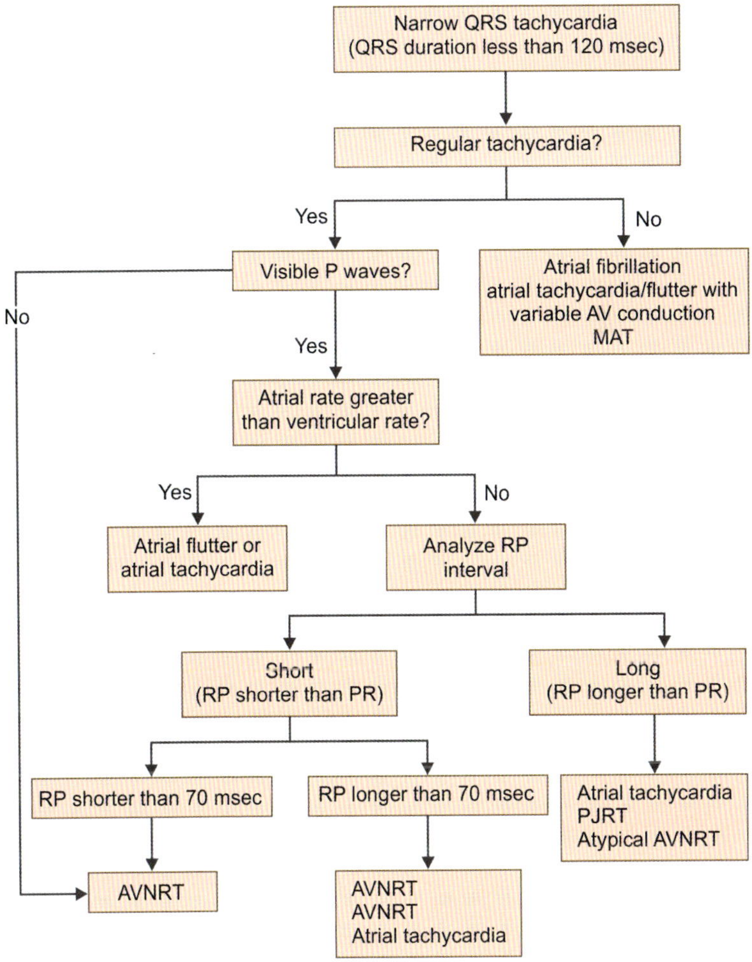

Algorithm for the diagnosis of a narrow-QRS tachycardia.

AVRT: Atrioventricular reentrant tachycardia; AVNRT: Atrioventricular nodal reentrant tachycardia; MAT: Multifocal atrial tachycardia; PJRT: Permanent form of AV junctional reciprocating tachycardia.

Focal Atrial Tachycardias (FAT)

Electrocardiographic Recognition

- Atrial rate (AR) – 150 to 250/min
- Very similar contours like normal P wave as they arise close to SAN.
- P wave usually in 2nd half of tachycardia cycle—i.e. long RP - short PR Tachycardia.
- If Atrial rate increases – AV conduction becomes Mobitz Type – 1 – 2 degree Heart block known as Atrial tachycardia with block.
- Nearly ½ of the cases AT with block, AR is irregular.

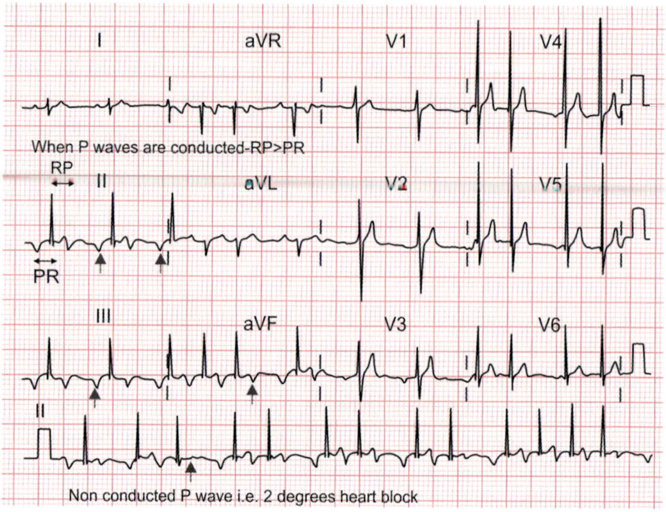

Note: PR and RP intervals in FAT.

MULTIFOCAL ATRIAL TACHYCARDIA (MAT) OR CHAOTIC ATRIAL TACHYCARDIA

- Commonly occurs in older patients with chronic obstructive pulmonary disease and congestive heart failure and may eventually develop into atrial fibrillation.
- Characterized by atrial rates between 100 and 130 beats/minute
- Marked variation in P wave morphology and totally irregular P-P intervals.

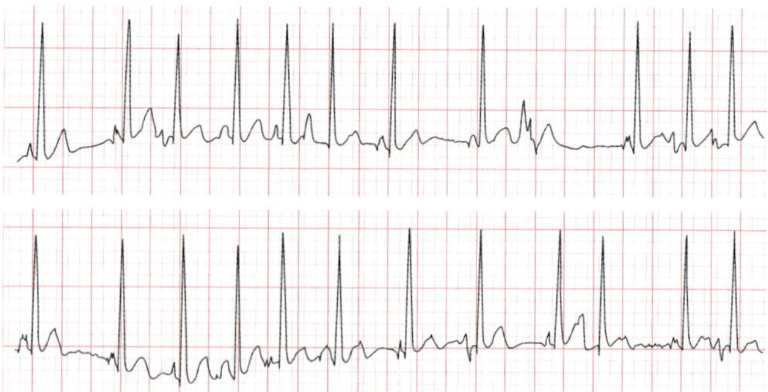

Chaotic (multifocal) atrial tachycardia. PACs occur at varying cycle lengths and with different contours.

Management

- **Potassium and magnesium replacement may suppress the tachycardia**.
- Avoid Beta blockers in patients with bronchospastic pulmonary disease but can be effective if tolerated.
- Verapamil and amiodarone have been useful.

17. Patient who is known case of thalassemia major already on repeated blood transfusions with history of iron overload previously treated with chelating agents. She came for BT now. During BT patient complained of backache and looks extremely anxious. What is next management?

a. Observe for a change in colour of the urine
b. Continue BT, do ECG
c. Stop BT and wait for patient to get normal and start
d. Stop BT and Do clerical check

Ans. d. Stop BT and Do clerical check

Classification and Etiopathogenesis of Transfusion Reaction

Acute Transfusion Reactions

- *Mild allergic reaction:* Attributed to hypersensitivity to a foreign protein in the donor product.
- *Anaphylactic:* More severe hypersensitivity reaction and sometimes related to IgA deficiency who makes alloantibodies against IgA and then receives blood products containing IgA.
- *Febrile non-hemolytic transfusion reaction (FHTR)*: Due to cytokines released from blood donor leukocytes (white blood cells).
- *Septic:* Caused by bacteria or bacterial by products (such as endotoxin).
- *Acute hemolytic transfusion reactions*: Immune-mediated reactions are often a result of recipient antibodies present to blood donor antigens.
- *Transfusion-associated circulatory overload (TACO):* Due to volume overload.
- *Transfusion-related acute lung injury(TRALI)*: Acute lung injury (non-cardiogenic pulmonary edema) is due to antibodies in the donor product (human leukocyte antigen or human neutrophil antigen) reacting with antigens in the recipient

Delayed Transfusion Reactions

- *Delayed hemolytic transfusion reaction*: Anamnestic response to a foreign antigen that the patient was previously exposed.
- *Transfusion-associated graft-versus-host disease*: Results from engraftment of donor lymphocytes (commonly found in cellular blood products) into an immunocompromised recipient's bone marrow. The donor lymphocytes recognize the patient as foreign and react against the recipient's body. The patient's immune system is unable to clear the foreign lymphocytes. **This is rare but often fatal**.

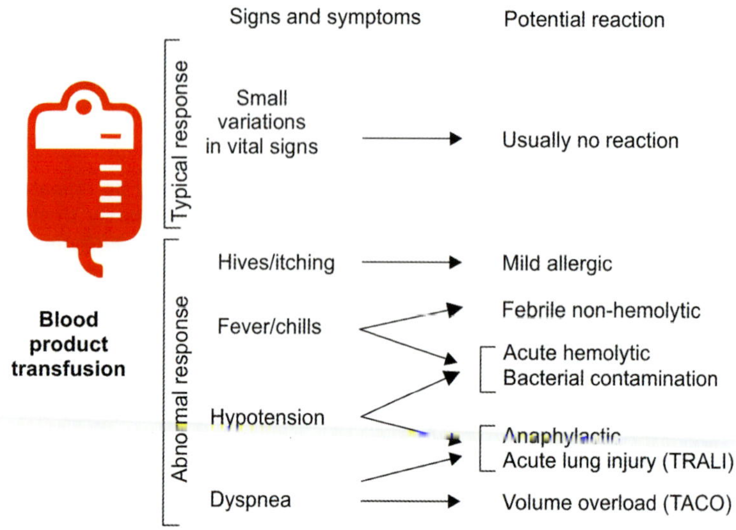

Summary

	Mild and common (1–4 in 100 units)		Severe and Rare (<1 in 5,000 units)		
	Febrile non-hemolytic transfusion reaction (FNHTR)	**Allergic reaction**	**Acute hemolytic transfusion reaction (AHTR)**	**Anaphylactic reaction**	**Transfusion-related acute lung injury (TRALI)**
Mechanism	Cytokine-mediated fever	Donor plasma proteins + recipient IgE→ mast cells activation → histamine release	ABO incompatibility →lysis of donor erythrocytes by preformed recipient antibodies	IgA-deficient patients release anti-IgA antibodies →histamine release	Donor antibodies + recipient leukocytes →leukocyte aggregation in pulmonary capillary bed
Signs and symptoms	Fever	Urticare, hives	Fever, tachypnea +/– flank pain and hemoglobinuria, DIC	Hypotension, angio-edema, respiratory distress	Respiratory distress
Time after transfusion initiated	1–6 hr	within 1 hr	Within 1 hr	Within minutes	Within 6 hr

Treatment	❑ Stop transfusion	❑ Pause transfusion ❑ Restart transfusion if symptoms resolve ❑ Antihystamines	❑ stop ransfusion ❑ Fluids and vasopressors if needed ❑ Mannitol if needed	❑ Strop transfusion ❑ Fluids and epinephrine ❑ Supposrtive care	❑ Oxygenation as needed ❑ Supportive

Two important first steps in any confirmed or suspected transfusion reaction are to

- ❑ Immediately stop the transfusion, and
- ❑ Contact the blood bank that issued the transfusion product.

18. Which of the following is *not* useful in measuring cardiac output?

a. Transthoracic echocardiogram
b. Central venous catheter
c. Thermodilution pulmonary catheter
d. Continuous cardiac output pulmonary catheter

Ans. b. Central venous catheter.

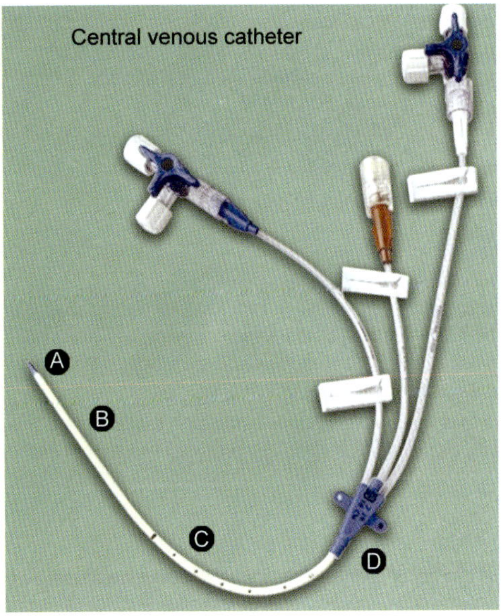

A central venous catheter is a catheter with a tip that lies within the proximal third of the superior vena cava, the right atrium, or the inferior vena cava. Catheters can be inserted through a peripheral vein or a proximal central vein, most commonly the internal jugular, subclavian, or femoral vein.

Indications for Central Venous Catheterization

- Access for drugs Infusion of irritant drugs—for example, chemotherapy.
- Poor peripheral access
- Long term administration of drugs, such as antibiotics
- Access for extracorporeal blood circuits
- Renal replacement therapy Plasma exchange
- **No role in cardiac output measurement.**

Monitoring or Interventions

- Central venous pressure
- Central venous blood oxygen saturation
- Pulmonary artery pressure
- Temporary transvenous pacing

Cardiac Output Measurements

- Cardiac output (Q) = SV x HR (L/min)
- A normal value of cardiac output at rest is about **4–8 L/min**.
- Cardiac index (CI) = SV x HR/BSA (L/min/m^2)
- **Normal Cardiac index = 2.5-4.2(L/min/m^2)**
- Stroke volume (SV) = end-diastolic volume – end systolic volume
- Ejection fraction (EF) = (SV/EDV) x 100%
- Normal EF—55%

Cardiac Output Measurement is done using Following Methods:

Cardiac output is estimated on various assumptions since no method is completely accurate. For comparison among patients, cardiac output is often corrected for the patient's size on the basis of body surface area and expressed as the cardiac index.

- Doppler echocardiography
- Dilution methods and especially thermodilution method
- Fick's principle, traditional method
- Non-invasive modifications of Fick's method

Doppler Echocardiography

- Stroke volume and that needs to be determined.
- **The volume(v)** flowing across a heart valve during one cardiac cycle. The volume that flows across a heart valve in any moment (*dV*) is equal to the duration of the moment (*dt*) multiplied by velocity of blood (*v*) and the cross sectional area of the valve (*A*).
- The total stroke volume is a sum of volumes that crossed the valve during all the moment of one cardiac cycle. Expressed mathematically:

$$dV = A \times v \times dt = \frac{\pi d^2}{4} v\, dt$$

SV = sum of all the *dVs* during one stroke

where *d* is the diameter of the valve (determined by echocardiography) and *v* is the velocity of blood determined by use of Doppler echocardiography.

Thermodilution Method

Cardiac output is measured by use of ***Swan Ganz catheter—pulmonary catheter***.

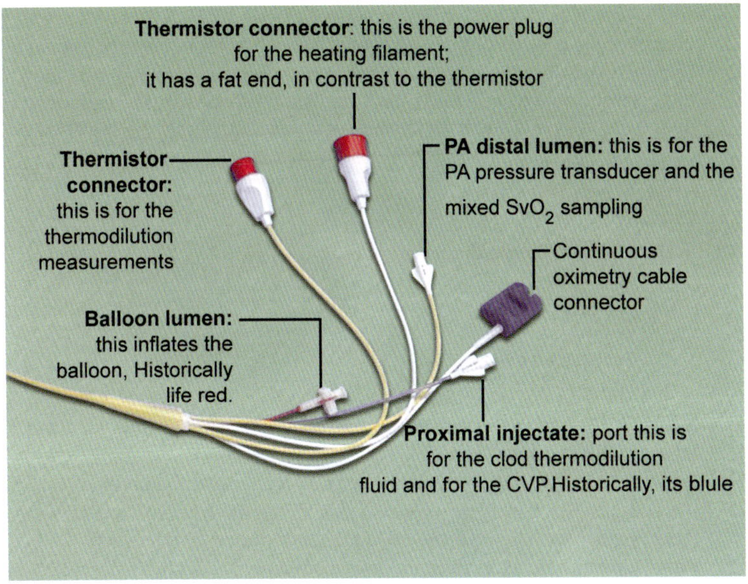
Thermistor connector: this is the power plug for the heating filament; it has a fat end, in contrast to the thermistor
Thermistor connector: this is for the thermodilution measurements
PA distal lumen: this is for the PA pressure transducer and the mixed SvO2 sampling
Continuous oximetry cable connector
Balloon lumen: this inflates the balloon, Historically life red.
Proximal injectate: port this is for the clod thermodilution fluid and for the CVP.Historically, its blule

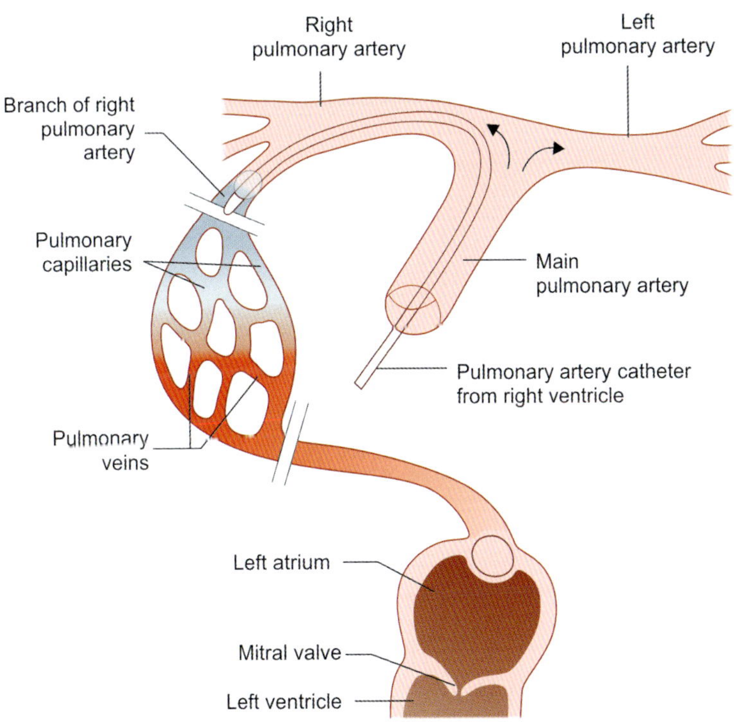
Right pulmonary artery
Left pulmonary artery
Branch of right pulmonary artery
Pulmonary capillaries
Main pulmonary artery
Pulmonary artery catheter from right ventricle
Pulmonary veins
Left atrium
Mitral valve
Left ventricle

Fick Method

- Fick principle is a straightforward application of the law of mass conservation.
- The difference between the (substance) amount of oxygen leaving lungs by arterial blood during one minute and the amount entering lungs by venous blood during same time is equal the amount of O_2 extracted from the breathed air.

Expressed by a Formula

$Q_{O_2\,Art} - Q_{O_2\,Ven} = Q_{O_2\,Air}$

19. Relative bradycardia is uncommon in:

a. Brucellosis
b. Typhoid
c. Malaria
d. Factitious fever

Ans: c. Malaria

- Relative bradycardia is an important diagnostic finding may be used to differentiate infectious diseases.
- Pulse-temperature relationships are based on physiological parameters.
- Physiologically, for each degree increase in temperature in degrees Fahrenheit, there is a commensurate increase in the heart rate of 10 beats/min.
- When temperature elevations are not accompanied by a physiologic increase in the pulse rate thus called ***pulse-temperature deficit***.

Determination of Relative Bradycardia Presented here in Table

Criteria	
Inclusive	
❑ Patient must be an adult, i.e. ≥13 years. ❑ Temperature ≥102 °F. ❑ Pulse must be taken simultaneously with the temperature elevation.	
Exclusive	
❑ Patient has NSR without arrhythmia, second/third-degree heart block or pacemaker-induced rhythm. ❑ Patient must not be on β-blocker medication.	
Appropriate temperature-pulse relationships	
Temperature	*Beats/min*
41.1 °f.f.s.C (106 °F)	150
40.6 °f.f.s.C (105 °F)	140
40.7 °f.f.s.C (104 °F)	130
39.4 °f.f.s.C (103 °F)	120
38.9 °f.f.s.C (102 °F)	120
38.3 °f.f.s.C (101 °F)	110

Note: Should only be applied to patients with temperatures in excess of 102°F.

Causes of Relative Bradycardia	
Infectious causes	
Intracellular organisms	
Gram-negative bacteria	*Salmonella typhi*
	Francisella tularensis
	Brucella spp.
	Coxiella burnetii (Q fever)
	Leptospira interrogans
	Legionella pneumophila
	Mycoplasma pneumoniae
Tick-borne organisms	*Rickettsia spp*
	Orientia tsutsugamushi (scrub typhus)
	Babesia spp.
Other	*Corynebacterium diphtheriae*
	Plasmodium spp. (malaria)
Viruses/viral infections	Yellow fever virus
	Dengue virus
	Viral hemorrhagic fevers
	Viral myocarditis
Noninfectious causes	Drug fever
	Beta blocker use
	Central nervous system lesions
	Malignant lymphoma
	Factitious fever

SURGERY

1. Patient with massive hemorrhage presents to the ER after RTA. What is not to be done?

a. Massive transfusion of fluid challenge
b. IV crystalloid 2L, within few minutes
c. Early tranexamic acid recommended
d. Check coagulation with thromboelastography, if available

Ans. b. IV crystalloid 2L, within few minutes (according to new ACLS protocol 2 liter is replaced by 1 liter)

- In fluid deficit management bolus dose of 1 liter lukewarm isotonic crystalline saline fluid is the standard protocol.
- Rest all are correct.

Important Points

a. Massive transfusion as per definition is of more than 10 units of blood in 24 hours or more than 4 units in 1 hour.
b. Tranexamic acid (TXA) reduces blood loss by inhibiting the enzymatic breakdown of fibrin. It is often used in surgery to decrease bleeding and the need for blood transfusion.
TXA (1 g loading dose over 10 min followed by an infusion of 1 g over 8 h) safely reduces mortality in bleeding trauma patients. Initiation of TXA treatment within 3 h of injury reduces the risk of hemorrhage death by about one-third, regardless of baseline risk. Because it does not have any serious adverse effects, TXA can be administered to a wide spectrum of bleeding trauma patients. Limiting its use to the most severely injured or those with a diagnosis of 'hyperfibrinolysis' would result in thousands of avoidable deaths.
c. Thromboelastometry is use to determine exact coagulation deficiency but available at only apex trauma centers.

Ref: Roberts I. Tranexamic acid in trauma: how should we use it? J Thromb Haemost. 2015 Jun;13 Suppl 1:S195-9. doi: 10.1111/jth.12878. Review. PubMed PMID: 26149023.

2. Following a RTA, a young man was brought to ER. Due to massive blood loss, 2 units of PRBC and 4 platelets obtained from blood bank. Only one IV line was accessible. What will you do?

a. Start PRBC 1st and store platelet at room temperature
b. Start platelet and store PRBC at room temperature
c. Only transfuse PRBC
d. Transfuse PRBC and store platelet at 2–6 degrees

Ans. a. Start PRBC 1st and store platelet at room temperature

- According to ATLS protocols PRBC is preferred over platelets. PRBC is supposed to transfuse within 4 hours of issue from blood bank otherwise cells lysis will start and hyperkalemia will occurs .
- Platelet can be stored at room temperature.

3. Patient had a RTA and put on mechanical ventilation, he is opening his eyes on verbal command, moves all his 4 limbs spontaneously. What will be his GCS score?

a. 12 b. 11
c. 9 d. 10

Ans. d. Ideally answers should be 9T/10 but not given in option then 10 is correct.

Since patient is intubated, have to use V_T instead of V_1.
Rest is E3M6.

4. A young patient has been admitted with RTA and had massive hemorrhage. He needs to be transfused with large amounts of fluids. Which IV cannula is preferred?

a. Grey b. Green
c. Blue d. Pink

Ans. b. Green (according to ACLS protocols two 18G cannula is sufficient in trauma patient)

Color	Gauge size	External diameter (mm)+	Length (mm)*	Water flow rate (ML/min)*	Recommended users
Orange 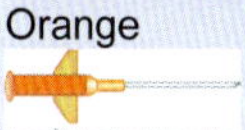	14G	2.1 mm	45 mm	–240 mL/min	Trauma, Rapid blood transfusion, Surgery
Gray 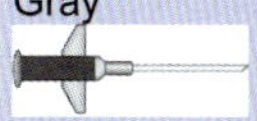	16 G	1.8 mm	45 mm	– 180 mL/min	Rapid fluid replacement, trauma, rapid blood transfusion
Green 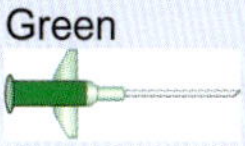	18 G	1.3 mm	32 mm	– 90 mL/min	Rapid fluid replacement, trauma, rapid blood transfusion
Pink 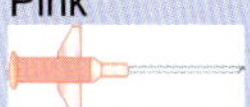	20 G	1.3 mm	32 mm	– 60 mL/min	Most infusion, rapid fluid replacement, Trauma, routine blood transfusion
Blue 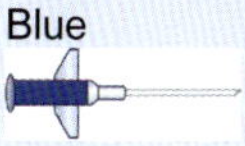	22G	0.9 mm	25 mm	– 36 mL/min	Most infusions, Neonate, pediatric, older adults routine blood transfusion
Yellow 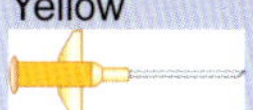	24 G	0.7 mm	19 mm	–20 mL/min	Most infusions neonate, pediatric, older adults, routine blood transfusion, neonate or pediatric blood transfusion
Purple 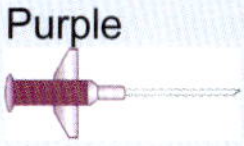	26 G	0.6	19 mm	–13 mL/min	Pediatrics, Neonate

5. A patient came with profuse diarrhea and dehydration reaches OPD. For examination flow of fluids which cannula can be inserted?

a. Green
b. Blue
c. Grey
d. Violet

Ans. c. Grey for rapid fluid replacement, Grey cannula has widest bore with flow rate of 180 mL/hr.

Rapid fluid replacement required in this patient.

6. While doing emergency laparotomy for an intestinal obstruction, which organ will you first visualize to say whether it is small bowel or large bowed obstruction?

a. Ileum
b. Sigmoid colon
c. Cecum
d. Rectum

Ans. c. Cecum: is always first to see in case of bowel obstruction.

- *Dilated cecum*: Large bowel obstruction
- *Collapsed cecum*: Small bowel collapse

7. What is the method of breast examination depicted in the video?

The clinician was palpating with tips of finger except thumb started from 2 O'clock posterior palpated at 3 points on line joining periphery to nipple. Then again went to 3 O'clock point directly and came back centripetally while palpating at 3 points again on the line joining periphery and nipple.

a. Vertical strip method
b. Concentric method
c. Clock wise method
d. Quadrant method

Ans. c. Clock wise method.

This method of examination is Dial clock/clockwise method.

- Examination was started at 12 O'clock position just below mid clavicular point and 6 O'clock being at infra-mammary crease.
- Palpation begin from periphery to the nipple by describing small circles of about 3 cm in diameter.
- Once nipple areola complex reached, next segment was palpated at 1 O'clock position.

8. Which is the most conspicuous sign in breast cancer?

a. Nipple retraction
b. Peau d'Orange
c. Puckering
d. Both nipple retraction and puckering

Ans. b. Peau d'Orange

Peau d'Orange is definitive sign of malignancy caused by infiltration of malignant cells in subdermal lymphatics.

- Nipple retraction can be seen in old age, fibrosis, previous retroareolar operative procedure.
- Puckering is seen in breast abscess.

9. What technique has been depicted in the image?

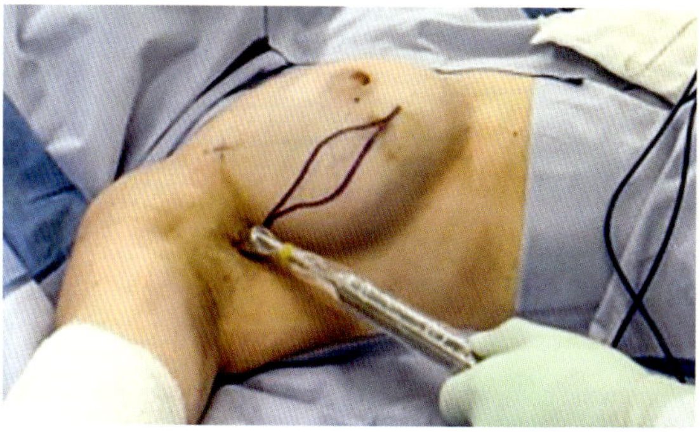

a. Brachytherapy
b. USG
c. Sentinel lymph node biopsy
d. Lateral pectoral nerve block

Ans. c. Sentinel lymph node biopsy

Procedure depicted in the figure is —Sentinal lymph node biopsy because:

- The probe shown in the figure is Gamma camera probe
- Above procedure is due to find out 1st draining axillary lymph node of breast mass.

10. Sentinel lymph node biopsy most useful for:

a. Ca cervix
b. Ca endometrium
c. Ca valva
d. Ca vagina

Ans. b. Ca Endometrium

Sentinel lymph node biopsy is most useful in Ca endometrium because:

- Detection rate of sentinel lymph node is 96% after cervical tracer injection.
- No intra-operative complications was associated.
- Reduction in average operative time
- Sentinel lymph node biopsy above resulted in a lower incidence of leg lymphedema.

11. Which flap-based procedure is used for pilonidal sinus surgery?

a. Rhomboid flap
b. Rotational flap
c. Free flap
d. Circular flap

Ans. a. Rhomboid flap

The procedure depicted in figure is rhomboidal flap because:

- A parallelogram shaped transposition flap is used to close the defect.
- Used in pilonidal sinus surgery
- It is a type of local flap

Next step is:

- Cessation of smoking —as it improve healing
- Do biopsy—incidence of malignant degeneration occurs in approx 0.1% of patients with recurrent pilonidal sinus.

12. The given below device is used for:

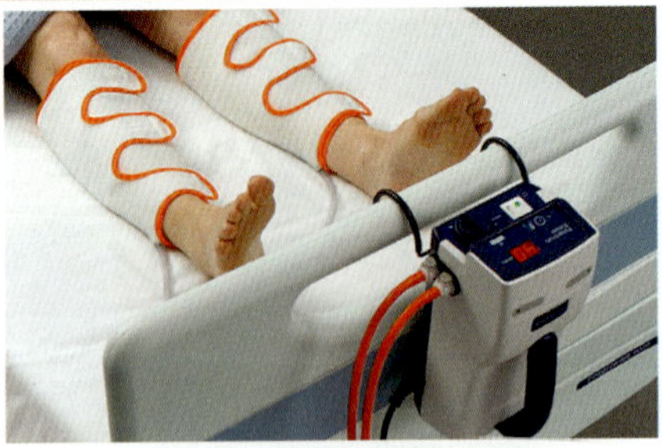

a. Pneumatic compression stocking to prevention of DVT
b. Varicose vein
c. Hypothermia
d. Cellulites

Ans. a. Pneumatic compression stocking to prevent DVT

Figure depicted above is intermittent pneumatic compression device used in:

- To prevent PVT
- Used in bed-ridden patient
- Contraindicated in acute DVT as chance of pulmonary embolism

13. The given instrument is used for harvesting the graft from healthy area in split skin thickness graft:

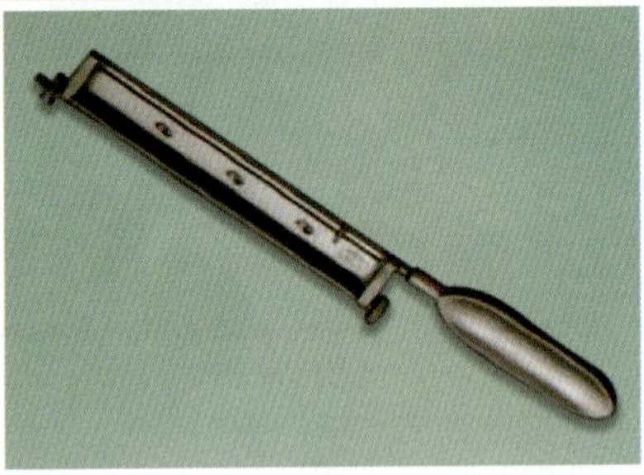

a. Dermatome
b. Silver's knife
c. Catlin amputating knife
d. Humby knife

Ans. d. Humby knife

Figure depicted above is:

- Humby's knife—used in split thickness skin grafting
- Thickness of graft can be adjusted by adjusting blades of knife.

b. Silver's knife

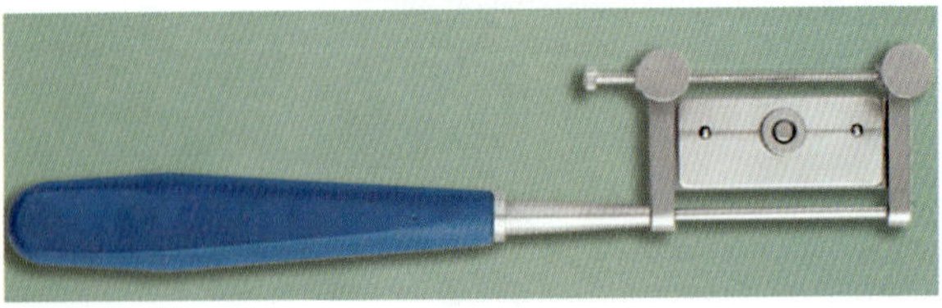

c. Catlin amputating knife

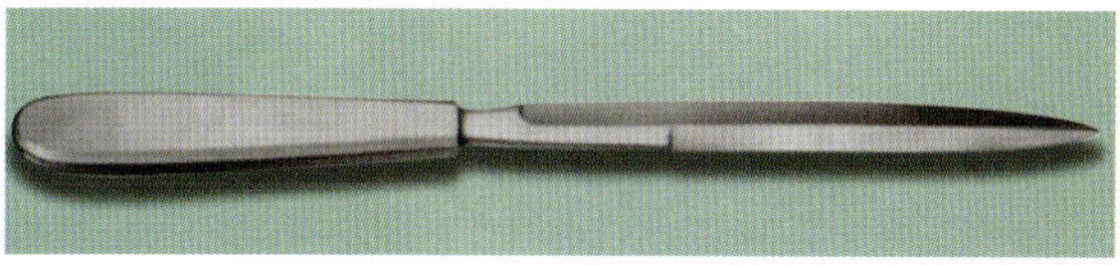

14. Name of the given instrument:

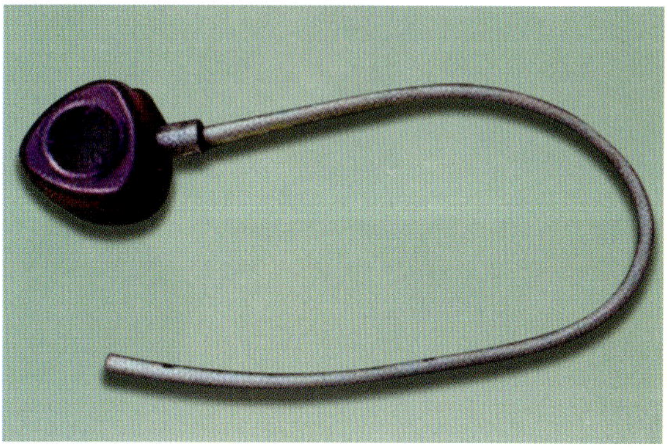

a. Gamma camera
b. Chemoport
c. IVC filter
d. Pacemaker

Ans. b. Chemoport

Figure depicted above is Chemoport

- Used in giving chemotherapy after MRM
- Generally inserted on contralateral side of chest of operative site.
- Decrease the requirement of cannulation each time giving chemotherapy, thus decreasing the risk of chemotherapy induced venous thrombosis.

Gamma Camera

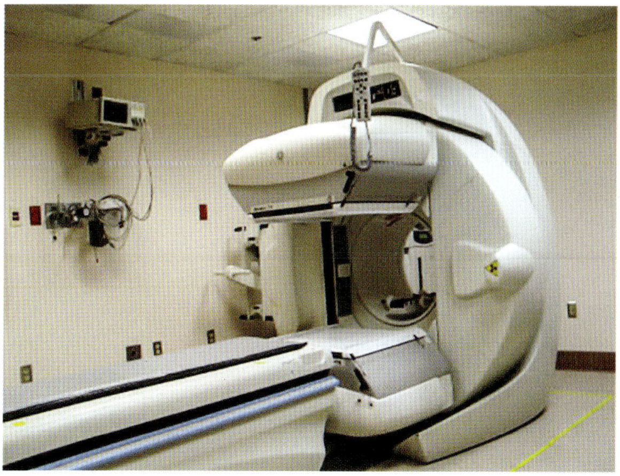

IVC filter

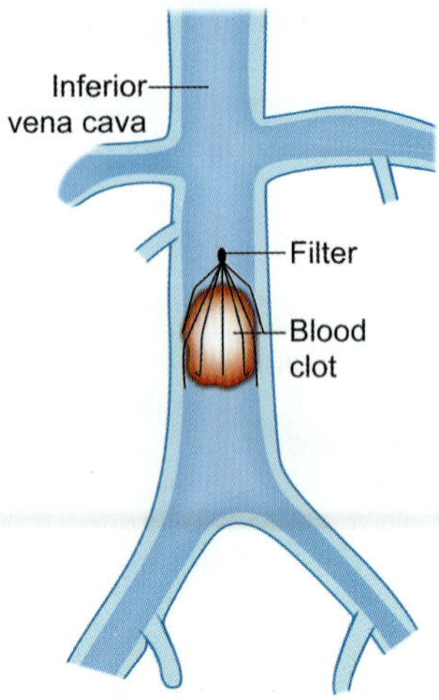

Indications

Relative indications include the following:

- Free-floating thrombus in the IVC or ileofemoral segments
- PE and limited cardiac reserve
- Prophylaxis in patients with severe traumas, spinal cord injury, or paraplegia
- Prophylaxis before surgery (in patients with DVT)
- Poor compliance with anticoagulation
- Protection during DVT thrombolysis

An absolute indication for IVC filter placement is the presence of DVT or PE with any of the following conditions:

- Contraindication for the anticoagulation
- Recurrent PE in spite of anticoagulation
- Anticoagulation-related complication

PEDIATRICS

1. Maximum steroid produced by fetal adrenal:

a. DHEA-S b. Cortisol
c. Corticosterone d. Progesterone

Ans. a. DHEA-S

- Shortly after the fetal adrenal gland forms (week 8-10), it efficiently secretes cortisol, which is able to negatively feedback on the fetal pituitary and hypothalamus to suppress ACTH secretion.
- This is critical time for differentiation of the external genitalia in both sexes; to prevent virilization, the female fetus must not be exposed to high levels of androgens of adrenal origin, and placental aromatase activity must remain low during this time to minimize conversion of testosterone to estradiol in male fetuses, which would interfere with masculinization.
- After week 12, HSD3B activity in the fetal adrenal gland decreases and steroid sulfokinase activity increases. Thus, the major steroid products of the mid gestation fetal adrenal gland are DHEA and DHEA sulfate (DHEAS) and, by 16α-hydroxylation in the liver, 16α-hydroxy DHEAS.

Ref: Nelson 19th edition, Ch.574

2. A 5-year-old boy has peculiar facial features, enlarged head, hepatosplenomegaly, protuberant abdomen, breathing difficulty with obstructive sleep apnea and cardiac valve thickening. What is the likely diagnosis?

a. Hurler's disease b. Hunter's disease
c. Fragile X syndrome d. Tay-Sachs disease

Ans. a. Hurler's disease

- Mucopolysaccharidosis are the result of intralysosomal accumulation of glycosaminoglycan fragments.
- Distended lysosomes accumulate in the cell, interfere with cell function and lead to characteristic pattern of clinical, radiologic, and biochemical abnormalities. Within this pattern, specific diseases can be recognized which evolve from the intracellular accumulation of different degradation products.
- As a general rule, the impaired degradation of heparan sulfate is more closely associated with intellectual disability.
- The impaired degradation of dermatan sulfate, chondroitin sulfates, and keratan sulfate with mesenchymal abnormalities.

Ref: Nelson 19th edition, Ch.88

Hurler Disease is autosomal recessive disease.

Present with Corneal clouding, mental retardation with death usually before 14 years of age. Dependent on severity of clinical presentation there are 3 types.

Severe Hurler, Hurler- Scheie and Scheie. Sheie present with corneal cloudind and aortic valve thickening.

Mucopolysaccharidoses				
Eponym	*Inheritance*	*Gene chromosome*	*Main clinical features*	*Defective enzvme*
Pfaundler-1-Hurler	AR	4p16.3	Severe Hurler phenotype, mental deficiency, corneal clouding, death usually before age 14 yr, Hurler phenotype, mental retardation, corneal clouding, death usually before age 14 yr	α-·L -iduronidase
Scheie	AR	4p16.4	Stiff joints, corneal clouding, aortic valve disease, normal intelligence, survive to adulthood	α-·L -iduronidase
Hurler-Scheie	AR	4p16.4	Phenotype intermediate between I-H and I-S	α-·L -iduronidase
Hunter	XLR	Xq27.3-28	Severe course similar to I-H but clear corneae. *Mild course*: less pronounced features, later manifestation survival to adulthood with mild or without mental deficiency	Iduronate sulfate sulfatase
Sanfilippo A	AR	17q25.3	Behavioral problems, sleeping disorder, aggression.	Heparan S-sulfamidase
Sanfilippo B	AR	17q21	Progressive dementia, mild dysmorphism, coarse hair,	N-Acetyl-α:-D-glucosaminidase
Hyaluronidase deficiency	AR	3p21.3	Periarticular masses, no Hurler phenotype H	Hyaluronidase 1

Hunter Syndrome

Is Autosomal recessive disease, presents with similar symptoms as Hurlers but clear cornea? Survival up to adulthood with or without mental retardation.

Tay Sach's Disease

Is GM2 gangliosidosis. Symptoms begin as early as 6 months of age with developmental delay and developmental regression with muscle weakness.

Fragile X Syndrome

Present with intellectual disability.

3. Which of the following is true statement regarding Turner's syndrome?

a. Turner syndrome with webbed neck is 3 times more likely to develop CVS defects than non-webbed neck
b. Coarctation of aorta is more likely in non-webbed neck
c. Male turner (Noonan syndrome) is much more likely to have CVS defects
d. Turner syndrome with webbed fingers and toes is likely to be associated with visceral anomalies

Ans. a. Turner syndrome with webbed neck is 3 times more likely to develop CVS defects than non-webbed neck

- Male turner is much more likely to have CVS defects because prevalence of pulmonary stenosis is 50% in Noonan and CVS defects prevalence in turners is overall 23% (PMID 9821430)
- *Turners:* 60% of infants with webbed neck is associated with CHD with high incidence of flow related defects such as hypoplastic left heart, coarctation of aorta and secundum arterial septal defects. 68% of infants with web neck had a genetic syndrome and 24% has dysmorphic feature consistent with lymphatic obstruction system.

4. BCG is maximally protective against:

a. Pulmonary TB
b. Pulmonary and CNS TB
c. CNS and disseminated TB
d. Extrapulmonary TB

Ans. c. CNS and disseminated TB (75 to 86% efficacy)

5. Video of a child having respiratory distress with audible grunting and asked about The Silverman Anderson Score:

(It is a video presented at a conference jointly held by AIIMS and PGI under The Queen Elizabeth Diamond Jubilee Trust and almost same video is available on YouTube and other resource forums.)

a. 7
b. 8
c. 9
d. 10

Ans. b. 8

- Silverman and Anderson's Score is used to know the severity respiratory distress in newborn children.

Feature	Score 0	Score 1	Score 2
Chest movement	Equal	Respiratory lag	Seesaw respiration
Intercostal retraction	None	Minimal	Marked
Xiphoid retraction	None	Minimal	Marked
Nasal flaring	None	Minimal	Marked
Expiratory grunt	None	Audible w/ stethoscope	Audible

6. A video of sick intubated neonate having bilateral jerks of both right and upper limbs with some occasional twitching of neck as well. Likely seizures:

a. Focal clonic
b. Multifocal clonic
c. Multifocal tonic clonic
d. Focal tonic

Ans. b. Multifocal clonic

What are Clonic Seizures?

These seizures cause rhythmic jerking movements (twitch like movement). When the rhythmic jerking movements are the only feature, it is a clonic seizure. These types of movements occur more frequently in association with a phase of muscle stiffening (see tonic-clonic seizures above). These seizures may also have a focal onset.

What are Tonic Seizures?

These seizures cause the muscles to stiffen. If a person is standing, a sudden increase in muscle tone could cause them to fall. Some people call this a **"drop attack"**. Generalized tonic seizures could also cause a sudden stiffening (or contraction) of the muscles in both arms. These seizures usually last less than 20 seconds, but sometimes they could be up to about 60 seconds. These seizures may also have a focal onset.

What are Focal or Generalized Atonic Seizures?

These seizures cause a loss of muscle tone, which means the individual suddenly becomes limp. If a person is standing, the sudden loss of muscle tone will cause them to fall. Therefore, both tonic seizures and atonic seizures can be associated with episodes that people may refer to as drop attacks.

These seizures may also have a focal onset.

Tonic- Clonic Seizures

In the **tonic** phase the body becomes entire rigid, and in the **clonic** phase there is uncontrolled jerking. **Tonic-clonic seizures** may or may not be preceded by an aura, and are often followed by headache, confusion, and sleep. They may last mere seconds, or continue for several minutes. Also known as a grand mal **seizure**.

Ref: Nelson 19th edition, Ch.593

7. Identify the instrument:

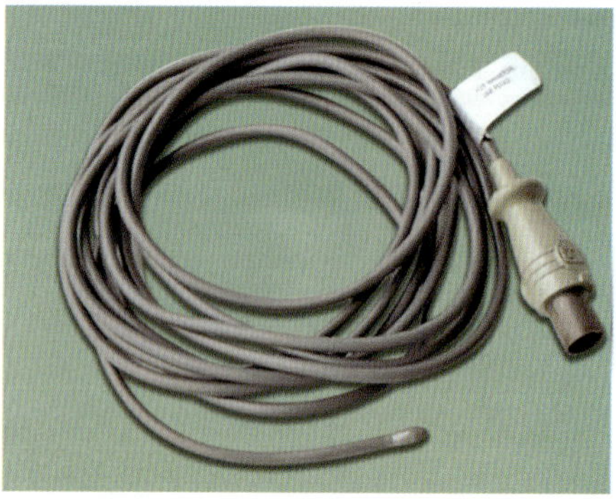

a. Swan Ganz catheter
b. NAVA catheter
c. Esophageal temperature probe
d. None of the above

Ans. c. Esophageal temperature probe

The Pulmonary Artery Catheter : Also known as Swan Ganz Catheter

The pulmonary artery catheter (PAC) is a balloon tipped thermo dilution catheter 110 cms long, that is inserted via a large vein and floated into the pulmonary artery. It is used to obtain hemodynamic measurements which together with clinical observations indicate how efficiently the heart is functioning.

The PAC directly measures:

- Right pulmonary systolic and diastolic pressures (PAP),
- Pulmonary artery wedge pressure (PAWP),
- Cardiac index (CI),
- Systemic and pulmonary vascular resistance (SVR & PVR),
- Core body temperature
- Mixed venous oxygen saturation.

These will be discussed later in this package

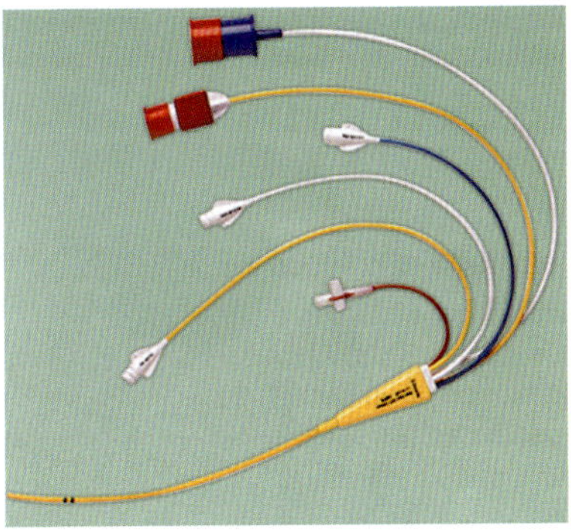

Nava catheter: (Neutrally adjusted ventilator assist)

- Neurally adjusted
  - Utilizes a catheter to detect the electrical activity signalling in the diaphragm Edi
  - Uses the strength of the Edi to determine how much assist to deliver to the patient
  - Bases each breath on the electrical signal, not trending from previous breaths

Esophageal Temperature Probe

It is used to measure the core body temperature.

OBSTETRICS AND GYNECOLOGY

1. Which of the following is not in quadruple test for antenatal detection of Down syndrome?

a. AFP
b. β-hCG
c. Estradiol
d. Inhibin B

Ans. d. Inhibin B

- **Quadruple test** is the second trimester measurement of maternal serum
- Alpha fetoprotein (MSAFP)
- Unconjugated estriol
- hCG
- Inhibin-A

It is done between 15–20 weeks.

	MS-AFP	Estriol	Inhibin A	β-hCG
Trisomy 18	↓	↓	↓	↓
Trisomy 21	↓	↓	↑	↑

2. Maternal mortality ratio expressed in:

a. Maternal death per 10,000 lives
b. Maternal death per 100,000 lives
c. Maternal death per 1,000,000 lives
d. Maternal death per 100 lives

Ans. b. Maternal death per 100,000 lives

$$MMR = \frac{\text{No. of maternal deaths}}{\text{Total number of live births}} \times 100{,}000$$

3. Dose of levonorgestrel used for emergency contraception:

a. 1–3 mg within 72 hours
b. 1.5 mg within 72 hours
c. 1.5 μg within 72 hours
d. 3 μg within 72 hours

Ans. b. 1.5 mg within 72 hours

- *For emergency*: 1.5 microgram in 2 doses within 72 hours.
  - Levonorgestrel given 0.75 mg in 2 doses within 72 hours of intercourse

4. A 55-year-old postmenopausal lady with simple endometrial hyperplasia with atypia. What is the management?

a. Hysterectomy
b. Mirena
c. Progestin
d. Estrogens

Ans. a. Hysterectomy

- Women with atypical hyperplasia should undergo a total hysterectomy because of the risk of underlying malignancy or progression to cancer.

- A laparoscopic approach to total hysterectomy is preferable to an abdominal approach as it is associated with a shorter hospital stay, less postoperative pain and quicker recovery.
- There is no benefit from intraoperative frozen section analysis of the endometrium or routine lymphadenectomy.
- Postmenopausal women with atypical hyperplasia should be offered bilateral salpingo oophorectomy together with the total hysterectomy

5. A 40-year-old female was diagnosed with CIN-3. What will be the management?

a. Trachelectomy
b. Hysterectomy
c. Conization
d. Colposcopy + LEEP

Ans. b. Hysterectomy

Risk factors for CIN: Young age at first intercourse (< 16 years)

Multiple Sexual Partners

- Cigarette smoking
- High parity
- Low socioeconomic status
- HPV infection
- Immunosuppression

Treatment options for CIN II and III are:

- LEEP/LLETZ in young patients who are desirous of future childbearing.
- If the patient is old or family is complete then this is treated by simple hysterectomy
- Option c & d are for 1A1 ca cervix in young women desirous of further childbearing.

CIN II and III require treatment in woman older than 21 year old.

The loop electrosurgical excision is a valuable tool for the diagnosis and treatment of CIN. It offers advantage of performing an operation that is simultaneously diagnostic and therapeutic during outpatient visit.

6. All of the following are reversible long acting contraceptives *except*:

a. Copper T
b. Laparoscopic tubal ligation
c. LNG- IUS
d. Implanon

Ans. b. Laparoscopic tubal ligation

- Laparoscopic tubal ligation is a surgical sterilization procedure in which a woman's fallopian tubes are either clamped and blocked or severed and sealed. Both methods prevent eggs from being fertilized. Tubal ligation is a permanent method of sterilization.

7. Possible cause of choriocarcinoma after hydatidiform mole is all *except*:

a. Rising hCG
b. More Theca lutein cysts
c. Increase uterus size
d. Suburethral nodule

Ans. d. Suburethral nodule

Suburethral Nodule is an unusual indicator of postmolar choriocarcinoma. All others are very well seen in the conversion of a complete hydatidiform mole into choriocarcinoma.

- Suburethral nodule may be a manifestation of vaginal metastasis from choriocarcinoma.
- Metastatic choriocarcinoma is however seen in only about 4% of patients after evacuation of a complete mole and vaginal metastasis that may present with suburethral nodule occur in only 30% of patients with such metastatic disease. Hence it is an unusual indicator.
- Raised β-hCG level present in choriocarcinoma

8. What should be the time of termination of pregnancy of a female with insulin dependent diabetes?

a. 40 weeks
b. 38 weeks
c. 37 weeks
d. 34 weeks

Ans. b. 38 weeks

- Pre-gestational/gestational diabetes with insulin requirement: terminated beyond 38 weeks
- Pre-gestational/gestational diabetes controlled on diet: can continue till 40 weeks

9. Active management of third stage of labor includes *except*:

a. Ergometrine after anterior shoulder delivery
b. Uterine massage
c. Cord traction
d. Oxytocin infusion

Ans. b. Uterine massage

Uterine massage is not a core component of Active Management of Third Stage of Labor (AMTSL).

AMTSL recommended by WHO is a triad including:

- Immediate administration of prophylactic uterotonic (Oxytocin)
- Controlled cord traction during placental delivery
- Delayed cord clamping

10. Investigation of choice for vesicovaginal fistula is:

a. IVP
b. Cystoscopy
c. 3 swab test
d. X-ray

Ans. c. 3 swab test

3 Swab Test (Vaginal Gauze Test)

- Three separate sponge swabs are placed into the vagina one above the other
- The bladder is them filled with a coloured agent such as methylene blue, and the swabs are removed after 10 minutes

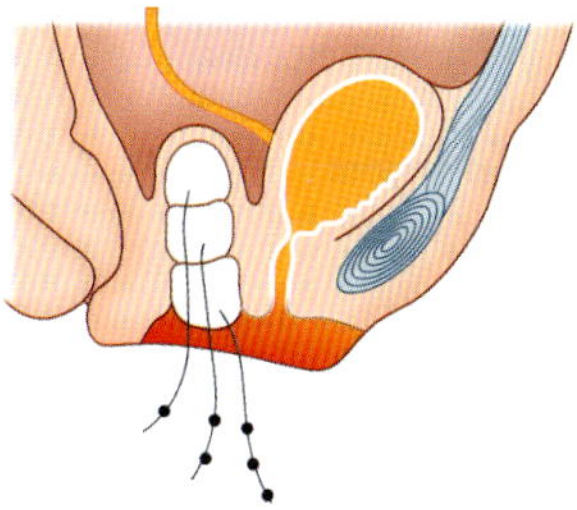

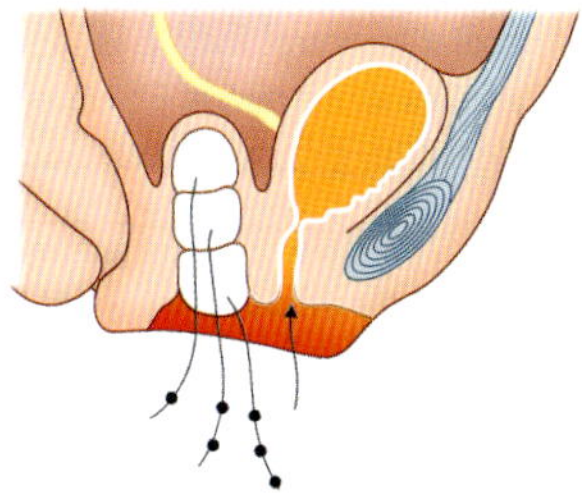

Results of 3 swab test

❑ Discolouration of topost swab is caused by vesico-veginal fistula	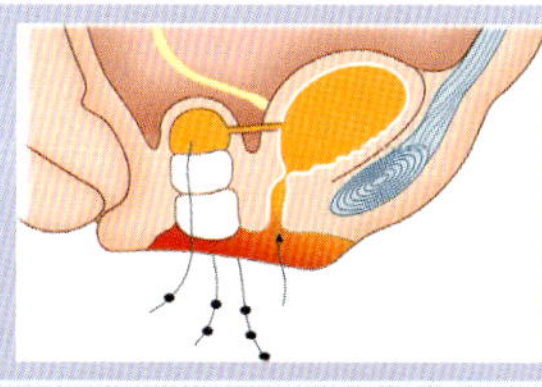
❑ Uppermost swab wetting but not discolouration suggest ureterovaginal fistula	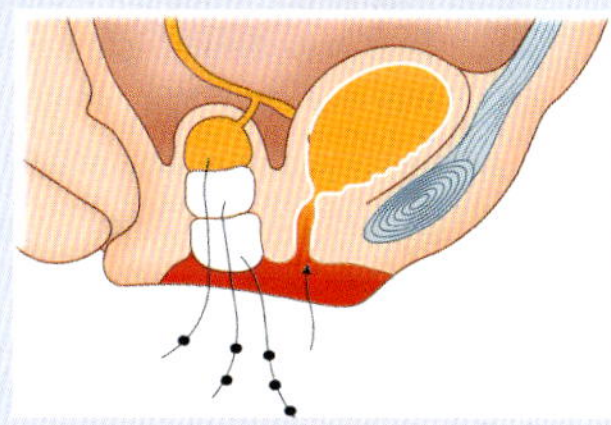
❑ Discolouration of only the lowest swab suggests low urethral fistula or from back flow into the introitus.	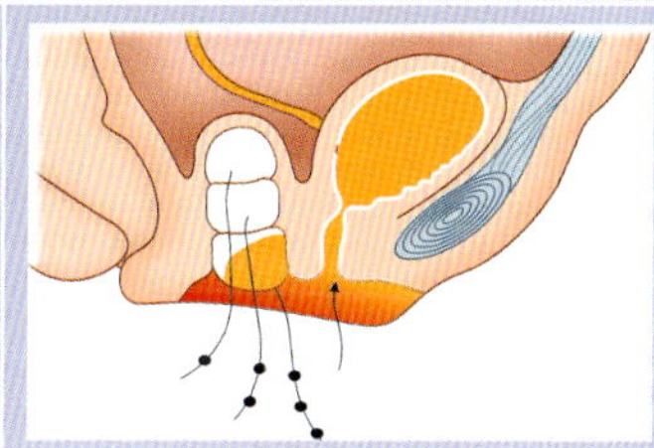

The investigations which are usually done in such cases are as follows:

- ❑ Urine culture
- ❑ Sonography of kidney, bladder and ureter
- ❑ IVP
- ❑ Cystoscopy with indigo carmine excretion test
- ❑ Methylene blue swab test

11. Before ovulation development of granules in a cell is dependent on:

a. Estrogen b. Progesterone
c. FSH d. LH

Ans. c. FSH

- Initial phase of follicular development before enter in menstrual cycle i.e. from primordial to antral follicle is independent of gonadotropins.
- Early follicular phase is FSH dependent
- Late follicular phase is both FSH and LH dependent

12. Young female history spontaneous abortion and secondary amenorrhea since then. FSH 6 IU/mL. What is the most probable cause of amenorrhea?

a. Ovarian failure
b. Pituitary failure
c. Fresh pregnancy
d. Uterine synechiae

Ans. d. Uterine synechiae

Since the lady in the question is having secondary amenorrhea following an abortion, uterine synechiae is the most likely cause.

Low normal FSH level is consistent with uterine abnormality. (Normal serum FSH value in adult woman is 5–20 IU/mL).

13. Placenta grade 3, 35+3 weeks pregnancy, and absent end diastolic flow in Doppler; next management is:

a. Dexamethasone and terminate after 48 hours
b. Terminate after 37 weeks
c. Talk with pediatrician and termination
d. Monitor and do nothing

Ans. c. Talk with pediatrician and termination

- *Absent end diastolic flow*: Fetal compromise (hence terminate pregnancy by cesarean section if >34 weeks)
- *Reverse end diastolic flow*: Impending doom of death (terminate pregnancy irrespective of gestational age).
- Steroids are given if pregnancy <34 weeks

DERMATOLOGY

1. What is the management for the given case?

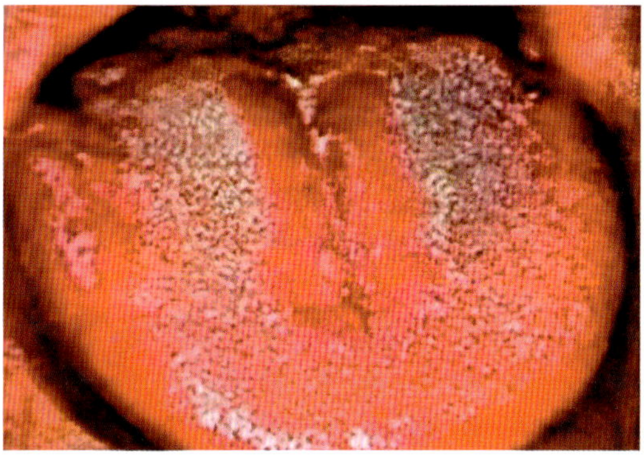

a. Dapsone plus steroids
b. Stop smoking and screen for carcinoma.
c. Vitamin supplements
d. Antifungals treatment for oral candidiasis

Ans. d. Antifungals treatment for oral candidiasis

- Median rhomboid glossitis
- Caused by Candida albicans
- *Treatment*: Antifungals

It is not erythroleukoplakia, so no screening for cancer required or associated with smoking

It is not the glossitis associated with vitamin deficiency which shows smooth bald tongue or large geographic areas of atrophy of the filiform papillae. This is not aphthous ulcer either.

It is not pemphigus (and so, treatment is not dapsone plus steroids) because pemphigus has superficial erosions only, while the photograph has a median erosion and peripheral white plaques.

2. A patient with history of bullae involving >30% BSA along with rashes all over body wlth erosions of the lips and other mucosa for few days. What can be the triggering factor?

a. Bacterial infection
b. Viral infection
c. Drug induced
d. Idiopathic

Ans. c. Drug induced

- History points to Toxic Epidermal Necrolysis (30% BSA, as opposed to SJS which is less than 10% BSA).
- The most common trigger for SJS-TEN is Drug induced more than viral etiology. (If this were erythema multiforme, the answer would be Virus > drug induced.)

Important Point:
SJS: When BSA involvement is <10–15%
SJS–TEN overlap: When BSA involvement is 10–30%
TEN: When BSA involvement is > 30%.

3. Identify the disorder with histopathology as shown in the figure.

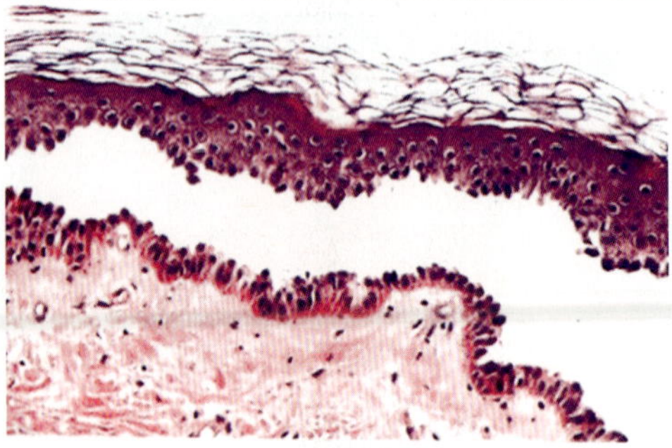

a. TEN
b. Lepromatous leprosy
c. Pemphigus vulgaris
d. Mycosis fungoides

Ans. c. Pemphigus vulgaris

- The biopsy shows a suprabasal split, with row-of-tombstones appearance of the basal layer of epidermis, and acantholytic cells are seen within the split.
- These are suggestive of Pemphigus Vulgaris.
- TEN has necrotic basal keratinocytes resulting in a split.
- Lepromatous Leprosy and mycosis fungoides have an almost normal epidermis, no split.

4. A 28-year-lady has asymptomatic dome-shaped small lesions on forehead for past 2 months. She lives with her 2 years old daughter, also having similar lesions. What is the causative agent of the lesions?

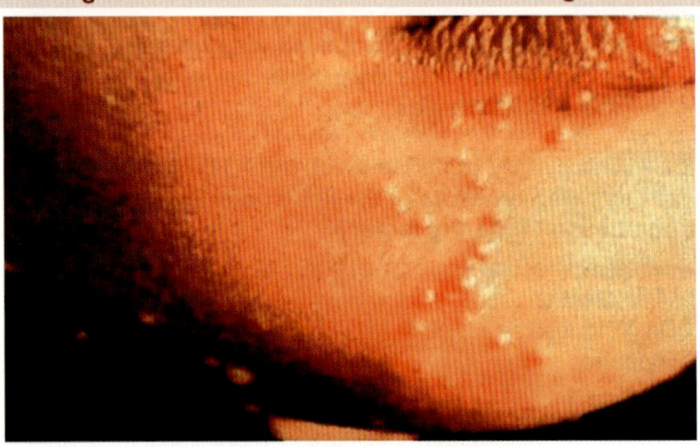

a. HSV
b. Poxvirus
c. HPV
d. VZV

Ans. b. Poxvirus

- The lesions are of molluscum contagiosum, thus the answer is Poxvirus.
- HSV causes herpes genitalis/labialis which are vesicular lesions/erosions, while molluscum contagiosum are dome-shaped, solid lesions. These are more common on face, usually occur in children or adults who are in close contact with young children.
- In this picture, the lesions below lip also appear to have a central umbilication - another feature of molluscum contagiosum.
- *HPV*: Papillomatous lesions
- *Chicken pox*: Single vesicles on erythematous base, trunk more than face

5. Patients with rashes in groin region as shown in the figure below. Which of the following cannot be the cause?

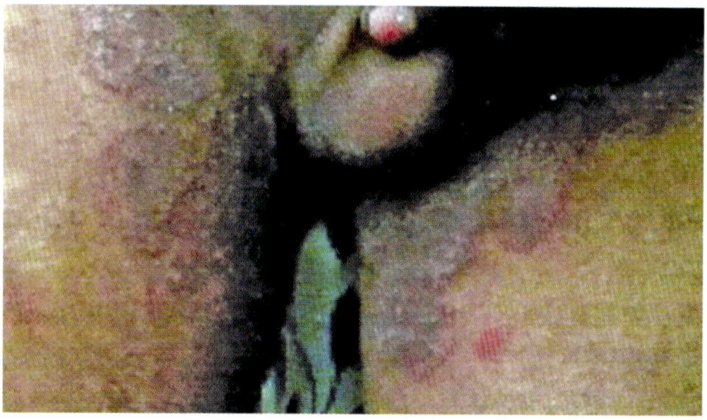

a. Aspergillus
b. Microsporum
c. Epidermophyton
d. Trichophyton

Ans. a. Aspergillus

- Erythematous, annular scaly plaques in bilateral groin suggestive of Dermatophytic infection.
- Aspergillus is not one of the dermatophytes, so answer is aspergillus.

6. Patients with 1 year history of painful nodulocystic acne as shown in the figure. What is drug of choice for the case?

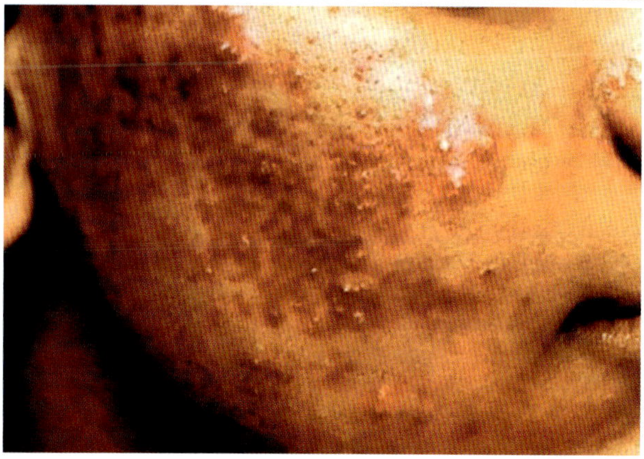

a. Topical clindamycin
b. Oral isotretinoin
c. Topical adapalene
d. Oral doxycycline

Ans. b. Oral isotretinoin

Drug of choice for painful nodulo-cystic acne is Oral Retinoids. Topicals are not helpful in this stage of Acne.

Principles of treating acne					
	Mild		Moderate		Severe
	Comedonal	Papulo-pustular	Papulo-pustular	Nodular	Nodular/ Conglobata
Drug of choice	Topical R	Topical R + Topical Ah/ BP	Oral Ab + Topical R + BP	Oral R	Oral Ab + Topical R + BP
Mainte-nance	Topical R	Topical R	Topical R	Topical R	Topical R
Females	–	–	–	Oral AA + topical R Oral R under supervision	Oral AA + topical R Oral R under Supervision

R: retinoids; Ab: antibiotics; BP: benzoyl peroxide, AzA: azelaic acid; AA antiandrogens

7. A child patient comes to OPD with history of black central arch rashes on his body, what is your diagnosis?

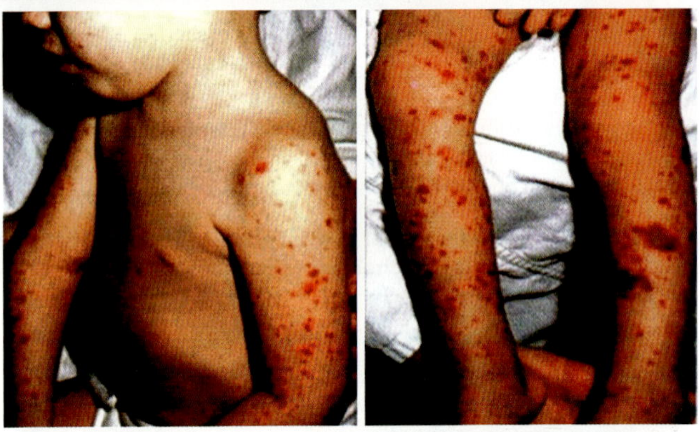

a. Meningococcemia
b. Dengue hemorrhagic fever
c. Leptospirosis
d. Scrub thypus

Controversial Question

- If the picture showed central eschar, then scrub typhus is the answer.
- However, if these are petechial and purpurin lesions, the answer is dengue.
- Meningococcal meningitis has confluent purpurae with a sick child.

1. Technique for Ryle's insertion:

a. Supine with neck flexed
b. Sitting with neck flexed
c. Supine with neck extended
d. Sitting with neck extended

Ans. b. Sitting with neck flexed

- Examine the patient's nostril for septal deviation. To determine which nostril is more patent, ask the patient to occlude each nostril and breathe through the other.
- Estimate the length of insertion by measuring the distance from the tip of the nose, around the ear, and down to just below the left costal margin. This point can be marked with a piece of tape on the tube. Nose-to-ear-to-xiphisternum (NEX) method.
- Position the patient sitting upright with the neck partially flexed. Ask the patient to hold the cup of water in his or her hand and put the straw in his or her mouth.
- Gently insert the NG tube along the floor of the nose, and advance it parallel to the nasal floor (i.e. directly perpendicular to the patient's head, not angled up into the nose) until it reaches the back of the nasopharynx, where resistance will be met (10–20 cm). At this time, ask the patient to sip on the water through the straw and start to swallow (see the image below). Continue to advance the NG tube until the distance of the previously estimated length is reached.
- If, at any time, the patient experiences respiratory distress, is unable to speak, or has significant nasal hemorrhage, or if the tube meets significant resistance, stop advancing the tube and withdraw it completely.
- Verify proper placement of the NG tube by auscultating a rush of air over the stomach using the 60 mL Toomey syringe (see the first image below) or by aspirating gastric content. The authors recommend always obtaining a chest radiograph.

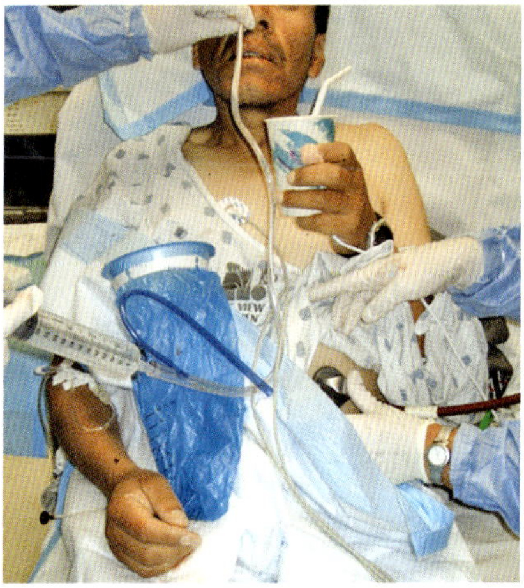

Ref: Medscape nasogastric intubation technique.

2. Which of the following statement is correct regarding difference between adult and child resuscitation?

a. Ventricular dysrhythmias are uncommon in children
b. Infant myocardium more refractory to hypoxia because of congenital heart disease.
c. More ventilation to be given compared to chest compression
d. Dissolved aortic oxygen concentration is more in pre-attack state

Ans: a. Ventricular dysrhythmias are uncommon in children

Like adults ventricular dysrhythmias are uncommon in children. Children experience cardiorespiratory attack secondarily and rarely as result of a primary cardiac event. This approach is critical because ACLS interventions primary directed toward the restoration of cardiac function may causes the physician to delay properly directed therapy, e.g. progressive respiratory failure with worsening hypoxia and respiratory acidosis leads to bradycardia and hypotension that can further progress to cardiac arrest

Ref: Page 3208 Miller's anaesthesia.

Why not

Ventilation to chest compression ratio is same in adult and children's, however children require smaller breaths than for adults (enough to make chest rise).

Dissolved low oxygen can present in pre-attack state.

RADIOLOGY

1. Which of the following is not ionizing radiation?

a. CT
b. MRI
c. Mammography
d. Angiography

Ans. b. MRI

- X-rays produced by X-ray tubes are used in CT scanners, X-ray crystallography, material and structure analysis.
- *Fluoroscopy*: Uses X-rays to obtain real time imaging
  - Used in interventional radiology
  - Image-guided surgeries
  - Diagnostic contrast studies.
- *Angiography*: To visualize the blood vessels after contrast injection using X-ray based techniques such as fluoroscopy.
- *Mammography*: Uses low energy X-rays (around 30 kVp) for screening and early detection of breast cancer
- *MRI*: Makes use of magnetic properties of nuclei

Ionizing radiation	Non-ionizing radiation
High energy radiation which can ionize an atom upon colliding with it to emit more radiation.	Non-ionising radiations are low energy radiations in which it does not emit particles from other materials.
High energy	Low energy
Can emit electrons or other particles from the atoms when they collide, e.g. Gamma rays, X-ray	Cannot emit particles from an atom, can only excite electrons from a lower level to a higher level upon encountering, e.g. UV, infrared, microwaves, radiowaves

2. Identify the given X-ray:

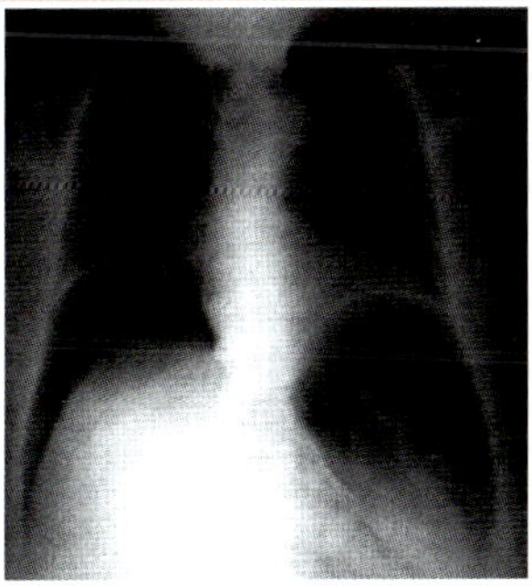

a. Pneumoperitoneum
b. Emphysema
c. Diaphragmatic hernia
d. Diaphragmatic eventration

Ans. a. Pneumoperitoneum

- Free air under diaphragm in erect Chest X-ray—pneumoperitoneum
- Diaphragmatic hernia

1. Bochdalek Hernia

- Most common fetal congenital diaphragmatic hernia
- Commoner on the left: 75–90%
- Posterolateral
- Large and associated with poorer outcome
- Presents earlier

2. Morgagni Hernia

- Less common
- Anterior
- Presents later

On Plain Radiograph

Indistinct diaphragm with opacification of part of or all the hemithorax (typically left sided)

- Scaphoid abdomen.
- Deviation of lines
  - Endotracheal tube
  - Nasogastric tube
  - Umbilical arterial and venous catheters

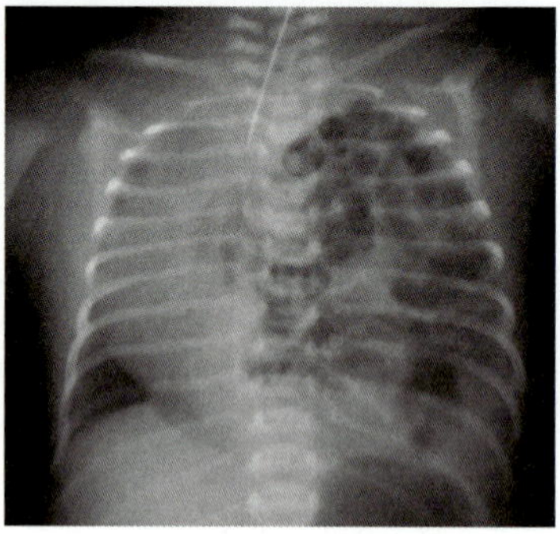

Emphysema

Except in the case of very advanced disease with bulla formation, chest radiography does not image emphysema directly, but rather infers the diagnosis due to associated features

- Hyperinflation
  - Flattened hemidiaphragm(s): most reliable sign
  - Increased and usually irregular radiolucency of the lungs
  - Increased retrosternal airspace
  - Increased anteroposterior diameter of the chest
  - Widely spaced ribs
  - Sternal bowing
  - Tenting of the diaphragm
  - Saber-sheath trachea

- Vascular changes
  - Paucity of blood vessels, often distorted
  - Pulmonary arterial hypertension
    - Pruning of peripheral vessels
    - Increased caliber of central arteries

Diaphragmatic Eventration

Elevation of the affected portion of the diaphragm is usually seen as a smooth hump, while the remainder of the hemidiaphragm contour is normal. The frontal X-ray may show a 'double' diaphragmatic contour, which is easily confirmed on the lateral projection.

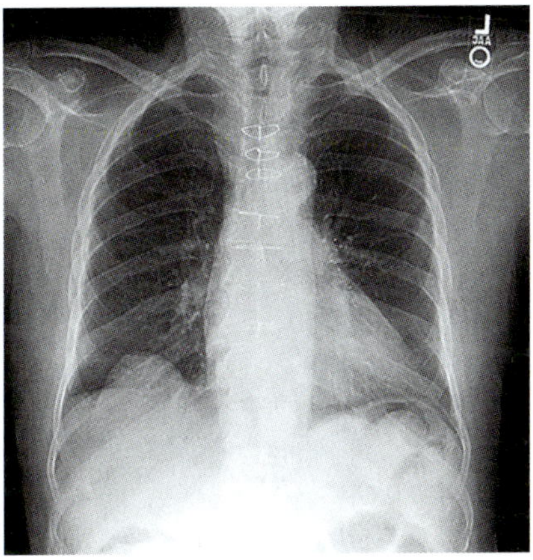

3. Empty Thecal sac sign in:

a. Arachnoiditis
b. Tethered Cord syndrome
c. Vertebral osteomyelitis
d. Discitis

Ans. a. Arachnoiditis

The *empty thecal sac sign or empty sac sign* is when the thecal sac appears empty on MRI of the lumbar spine, best seen on T2-weighted images. If the empty thecal sac sign is present, a diagnosis of adhesive arachnoiditis can be made.

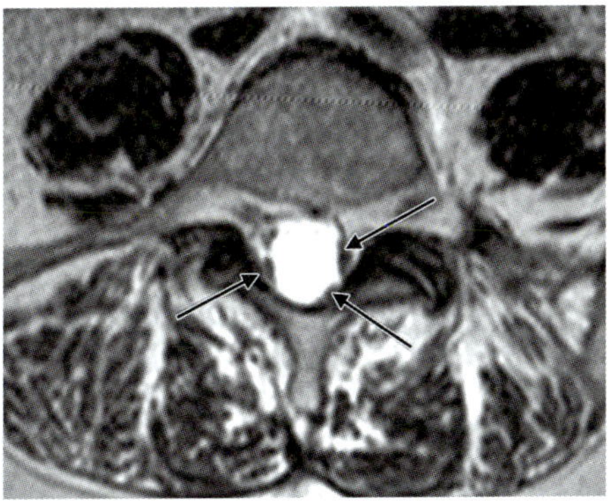

4. Identify the type of investigation done:

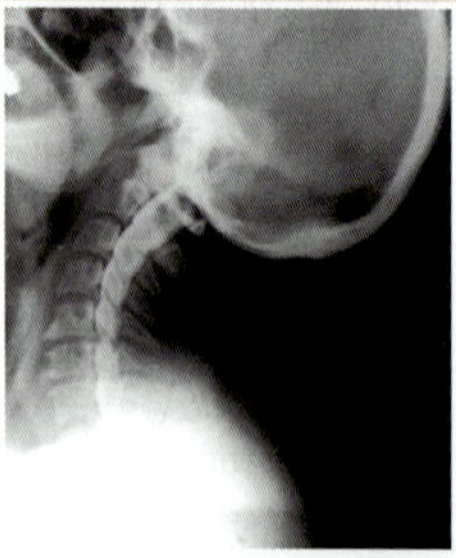

a. Angiography
b. Fluoroscopy
c. Myelography
d. Neurography

Ans. c. Myelography

Here you can see white structure between vertebral body and spinous process, so contrast in spinal canal is myelography.

5. Identify the given X-ray image:

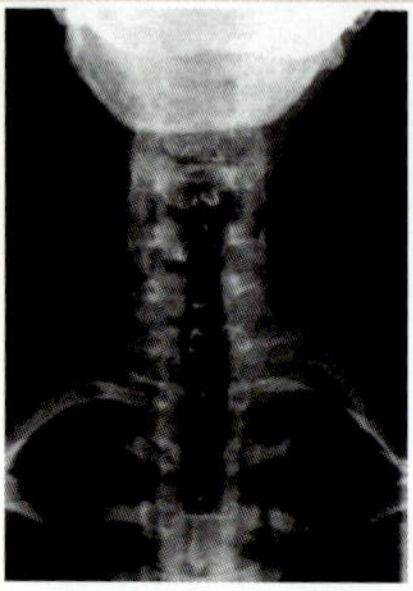

a. Cervical rib
b. Costochondritis
c. Fracture 2nd rib
d. Spondylolisthesis

Ans. a. Cervical rib

- Cervical rib arises from the seventh cervical vertebra.
- They occur in ~0.5% of the population, are usually bilateral, but often asymmetric
- More common in females
- Although cervical ribs are usually asymptomatic, they are the most important anatomic rib variant clinically, because they can cause thoracic outlet syndrome by compression of the brachial plexus or subclavian vessels.

Costochondritis

- Self-limited
- Usually multiple affected levels
- Multiple etiology
- Can occur at the costochondral junction or at the chondrosternal joints
- No swelling or induration on physical examination
- Pain that is reproduced by palpation and may radiate on the chest wall

Spondylolisthesis denotes the slippage of one vertebra relative to the one below. Spondylolisthesis can occur anywhere but is most frequent, particularly when due to spondylolysis, at L5/S1 and to a lesser degree L4/L5.

PSYCHIATRY

1. Provision of mental health Act 2017 based WHO mental health action gap programme are all, except:

a. Human rights
b. Communication regarding care and career
c. Screening family members
d. Social support

Ans. c. Screening family members

- Mental health gap action programme: Aim is to scale up services for mental neurological and substance use disorder (for low and middle income country)
- Scale up services for Mental, neurological and substance use disorders

Purpose

- Provide care
- Spread awareness
- Psychosocial assistance
- Building communication
- Giving medication

Principles Include

A. Universal health coverage
B. Human rights
C. Evidence based practices
D. Life course approach
E. Multisectoral approach
F. Empowerment of People with mental neurological and substance use disorder.

Ref: WHO mental health action gap programme.

2. SPIKES protocol is used for:

a. Triage
b. Communication with patients/attendants regarding bad news
c. Writing death certificate
d. RCT

Ans. b. Communication with patients/attendants regarding bad news

- Bad news may be defined as "any information which adversely and seriously affects an individual's view of his or her future"

The Six Steps of SPIKES

STEP 1: S—SETTING UP the Interview

Mental rehearsal is a useful way for preparing for stressful tasks. This can be accomplished by reviewing the plan for telling the patient and how one will respond to patients' emotional reactions or difficult questions. As the messenger of bad news, one should expect to have negative feelings and to feel frustration or responsibility. It is helpful to be reminded that, although bad news may be very sad for the patients, the information may be important in allowing them to plan for the future.

STEP 2: P—Assessing the Patient's PERCEPTION

Steps 2 and 3 of SPIKES are points in the interview where you implement the axiom "before you tell, ask." That is, before discussing the medical findings, the clinician uses open-ended questions to create a reasonably accurate picture of how the patient perceives the medical situation—what it is and whether it is serious or not. For example, "What have you been told about your medical situation so far?" or "What is your understanding of the reasons we did the MRI?". Based on this information you can correct misinformation and tailor the bad news to what the patient understands.

STEP 3: I—Obtaining the Patient's INVITATION

While a majority of patients express a desire for full information about their diagnosis, prognosis, and details of their illness, some patients do not. When a clinician hears a patient express explicitly a desire for information, it may lessen the anxiety associated with divulging the bad news.

STEP 4: K—Giving KNOWLEDGE and Information to the Patient

Warning the patient that bad news is coming may lessen the shock that can follow the disclosure of bad news. Examples of phrases that can be used include, "Unfortunately I've got some bad news to tell you" or "I'm sorry to tell you that…"

STEP 5: E—Addressing the Patient's EMOTIONS with Empathic Responses

Responding to the patient's emotions is one of the most difficult challenges of breaking bad news.

Patients' emotional reactions may vary from silence to disbelief, crying, denial, or anger.

An empathic response consists of four steps.

- First, observe for any emotion on the part of the patient. This may be tearfulness, a look of sadness, silence, or shock.
- Second, identify the emotion experienced by the patient by naming it to oneself. If a patient appears sad but is silent, use open questions to query the patient as to what they are thinking or feeling.
- Third, identify the reason for the emotion. This is usually connected to the bad news. However, if you are not sure, again, ask the patient.
- Fourth, after you have given the patient a brief period of time to express his or her feelings, let the patient know that you have connected the emotion with the reason for the emotion by making a connecting statement.

STEP 6: S—STRATEGY and SUMMARY

Patients who have a clear plan for the future are less likely to feel anxious and uncertain. Before discussing a treatment plan, it is important to ask patients if they are ready at that time for such a discussion. Presenting treatment options to patients when they are available is not only a legal mandate in some cases, but it will establish the perception that the physician regards their wishes as important. Sharing responsibility for decision-making with the patient may also reduce any sense of failure on the part of the physician when treatment is not successful. Checking the patient's misunderstanding of the discussion can prevent the documented tendency of patients to overestimate the efficacy or misunderstand the purpose of treatment

Ref: http://theoncologist.alphamedpress.org/content/5/4/302.long

3. An individual with a known psychiatric disorder or on treatment and is not a minor can chose to decide the care taker and the course of treatment according to mental health act. This is called:

a. Advance directive
b. Treatment directive
c. Mental will
d. Future directive

Ans. a. Advance directive

Advance Directive

- Every person, who is not a minor, shall have a right to make an advance directive in writing, specifying any or all of the following, namely:—
  - The way the person wishes to be cared for and treated for a mental illness;
  - The way the person wishes not to be cared for and treated for a mental illness;
- Person can also specify order of precedence, as he/she wants to appoint someone nominative representative.

Any person who is not minor has right to appoint nominative representative.

Nominative representative have right to make decision in absence of decision making capacity of person.

Order of Precedence

A. Individual appointed in the advanced directive as nominative representative.
B. Relative can be a nominative representative
C. Care giver can be a nominative representative
D. Suitable person appoint by concerned board
E. Board shall appoint the director of social welfare as nominative representative. Or anyone designative person can appoint as NR. Ref: mental health care act 2017